A Colour Atlas of

Optic Disc Abnormalities

Erna E. Kritzinger, MSc, FRCS, MRCP
Consultant Ophthalmologist,
Birmingham and Midland Eye Hospital,
Senior Clinical Lecturer in Ophthalmology,
Medical School, University of Birmingham,
Birmingham, England.

Heather M. Beaumont, BSc, PhD
Former Senior Lecturer in Embryology,
Department of Anatomy, Medical School,
University of Birmingham,
Birmingham, England.

Wolfe Medical Publications Ltd
Year Book Medical Publishers, Inc.

Copyright © Erna E. Kritzinger, Heather M. Beaumont, 1987
Published by Wolfe Medical Publications Ltd, 1987
Printed by W.S. Cowell Ltd, 8 Butter Market, Ipswich, England
UK ISBN 0 7243 0915 3

For a full list of other atlases published by Wolfe Medical Publications Ltd,
please write to the publishers at: Wolfe House, 3 Conway Street, London, W1P 6HE,
England *or* Year Book Medical Publishers, Inc., 35 East Wacker Drive, Chicago,
Ill. 60601, USA.

Distributed in Continental North America,
Hawaii and Puerto Rico by
Year Book Medical Publishers, Inc.

Library of Congress Cataloging in Publication Data

Kritzinger, Erna E.
    A colour atlas of optic disc abnormalities.

    Includes index.
    1. Optic disc—Abnormalities—Atlases.   I. Beaumont,
Heather M.   II. Title.   [DNLM: 1. Optic Disk—
abnormalities—atlases.   WW 17 K92ca]
RE728.067K75   1987   617.7′3   86-18964
ISBN 0-8151-5172-1

Contents

Acknowledgements

We are grateful to Dr Joseph B. Walsh (Montefiore Hospital; New York Eye and Ear Infirmary) for his advice and constructive criticisms and Dr D. C. Lea for her helpful comments on the manuscript; also to Mrs D. Thomas for assistance with the preparation of the diagrams.

We are indebted to the following for the figures listed below:

Dr W. H. P. Cant, Birmingham (17).

Miss M. M. G. Clover, Auckland, NZ (29, 32, 127).

Professor P. Henkind, New York (111).

Dr E. Nikoskelainen and Mr K. Nummelin, Turku, Finland (76, 77, 78).

Mr E. C. O'Neill, Birmingham (87).

Mr K. Rubinstein, Birmingham (23, 26, 38, 48, 103, 109).

Dr B. E. Wright, Keene, USA (37, 44, 45, 50, 73, 120, 122, 134, 135, 137).

Dr J. B. Walsh, New York (49, 69, 115, 118, 136).

Figure **77** is reproduced from Archives in Ophthalmology, 1983, Volume 101, Number 7, page 1064 (copyright 1983, American Medical Association).

Introduction

The purpose of this Atlas is to illustrate and describe abnormalities of the optic disc and to provide a practical guide to the recognition of those congenital and acquired disorders that affect it. Retinal abnormalities that are topographically related to the optic disc are also included. To assist differential diagnosis, all of the conditions appearing in the book are listed and categorized in a diagnostic key which is based on the ophthalmoscopic features of each abnormality.

Although, ideally, the fundus should be examined through a pupil that has been dilated, this is not always practicable. Nevertheless, the optic disc is usually visible on ophthalmoscopy, even through the undilated pupil. Thus ophthalmoscopic examination of the optic disc and surrounding retina offers important clues to diagnosis of the ocular condition. It may also provide indications for further investigation of the patient for an associated systemic disease.

This book is therefore designed as an aid to all who inspect the fundus ophthalmoscopically, especially those engaged in postgraduate studies in ophthalmology, internal medicine, paediatrics, or neurology, also general practitioners and opticians.

Erna E. Kritzinger
Heather M. Beaumont, 1986

Diagnostic Key

Based on Ophthalmoscopic Features

(References are to page numbers)

'Excavated' disc
Coloboma, 21
Optic disc pit, 26
Morning glory optic disc, 31
Myopia, 70
Glaucoma, 72
Avulsion, 74

Small disc
Hypoplasia, 28
Optic disc drusen (child), 81
Hypermetropia, 84

Pale, swollen and/or distorted disc
Myelinated nerve fibres, 34
Bergmeister's papilla, 37
Persistent hyperplastic primary vitreous, 40
Idiopathic ischaemic optic neuropathy
    (papillopathy), 61
Giant cell arteritis (Arteritic papillopathy),
    62
Secondary optic atrophy, 68
Papilloedema (longstanding), 75
Optic disc drusen (advanced), 81
Astrocytic hamartoma, 87
Glioma, 95
Meningioma, 97
Retinoblastoma, 98
Metastases, 104
Leukaemic infiltrates, 105
Granuloma (end stage), 107
Juxtapapillary choroiditis, 108

Pale and flat disc
Optic neuritis (retrobulbar neuritis), 59
Idiopathic ischaemic optic neuropathy
    (retrobulbar optic neuropathy), 61
Primary optic atrophy, 67
Consecutive optic atrophy, 68

'Enlarged' disc
Coloboma, 21
Optic disc pit, 26
Megalopapilla, 30
Morning glory optic disc, 31
Myelinated nerve fibres, 34
Myopia, 70

'Hyperaemic', swollen and/or distorted disc
Tilted disc, 24
Retinal vein occlusion, 51
Optic neuritis (papillitis), 59
Diabetic papillopathy, 63
Leber's hereditary optic neuropathy, 64
Papilloedema (including hypertension), 75, 79
Optic disc drusen (adult), 81
Hypermetropia, 84
Capillary haemangioma, 92
Granuloma (acute), 107

1: The Optic Disc

Ophthalmoscopy

The optic disc is the intraocular portion of the optic nerve, visible ophthalmoscopically; it marks the radial convergence of fibres from the neural retina and the point at which they exit from the eye. The alternative name, optic papilla, denotes the slightly elevated periphery of the disc. However, reference to the papilla is most often made in a descriptive context, either to designate peripapillary or juxtapapillary regions of the retina (thus defining a topographical relationship to the optic disc), or in the naming of pathological conditions, such as papilloedema and papillitis.

The term optic nerve head relates to the anterior portion of the optic nerve, lying within the scleral canal. It comprises not only the superficial optic disc or papilla, but also the underlying prelaminar layer of the optic nerve and the region of the lamina cribrosa (*see* below). The retrolaminar or retrobulbar portion of the optic nerve commences posterior to the lamina cribrosa and scleral canal.

General features

Viewed ophthalmoscopically, the optic disc appears circular or slightly ovoid in form (elongated in the horizontal axis); it is about 1.5 mm in diameter. The centre of the disc lies approximately 4 mm nasally and 1 mm

1 Normal fundus showing the optic disc lying superonasally in relation to the fovea (the vertical line is a foveal fixation target in the camera).

1

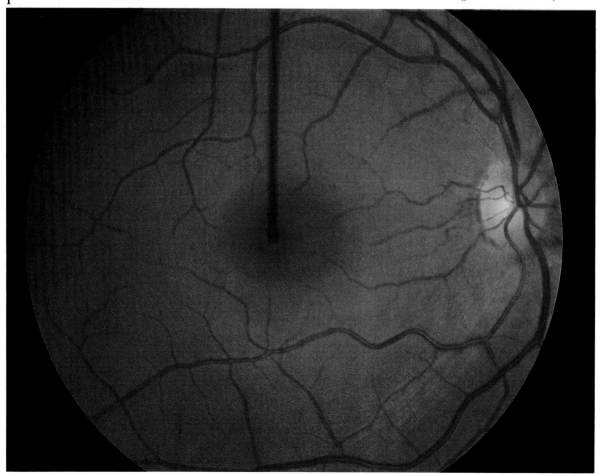

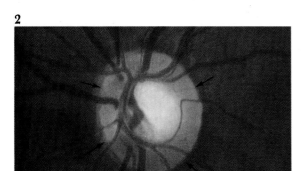

2 Normal optic disc showing distinct margin (arrows), pink neural rim and pale physiological cup.

3 Central retinal vessels emerging from the nasal side (arrows) of the physiological cup in a normal optic disc.

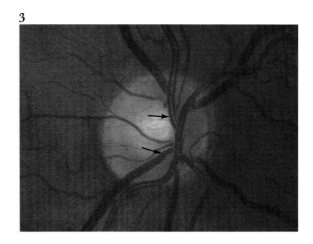

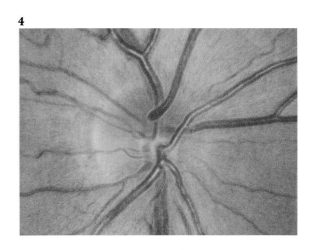

4 Small optic disc. The physiological cup is absent and the retinal vessels emerge centrally.

superiorly in relation to the fovea (Fig. **1**). Meridians transecting the optic disc at right angles are used, for the purpose of description, to divide the posterior fundus into four sectors, namely the superior and inferior nasal and temporal quadrants.

Features of the optic disc that are employed in clinical assessment and diagnosis include its colour and shape and the characteristics of the physiological cup, neural rim, margin of the disc and retinal blood vessels (Figs. **2** and **3**). Variations in the appearance of these elements may signify disease, or represent part of a wide spectrum of normality.

The outer portion, or neural rim, of the normal optic disc is yellow–pink in colour (although the temporal side is often paler than the nasal side), whereas the centre of the disc is occupied by a funnel-shaped depression— the physiological cup—almost white in appearance. Optic nerve fibres converge at the elevated neural rim, where they turn at right angles away from the retina and pass backwards towards the brain in the optic nerve. The pink coloration of the neural rim derives from its rich capillary network. In contrast, the cupped portion of the disc is relatively avascular and hence considerably paler; it consists chiefly of astrocytes and connective tissue.

There are variations in the size of the optic disc and physiological cup. In normal eyes the number of optic nerve fibres, and the area of neural rim which they comprise, is constant. Thus a small optic disc tends to have a small cup because of the concentration of nerve fibres at their point of confluence. Quantitatively, the diameter of the physiological cup is expressed as a ratio of the diameter of the disc, measured along the vertical axis. There is a wide variation in the cup:disc ratio in normal eyes (0.1–0.9) (Figs. **4** and **5**); the size of the cup may increase slightly with age.

The depth of the physiological cup also varies in normal eyes. Larger cups tend to be deeper so that, in about 30 per cent of eyes, the lamina cribrosa is revealed. This 'mesh' of connective tissue has a yellow–white sieve-like appearance, seen in the base of the physiological cup.

The parameter cup:disc ratio is important in the diagnosis and assessment of *glaucoma* (*see* page 72). In this condition the physiological cup increases in diameter, particularly along its vertical axis. This is correlated with a reduction in the neural rim, brought about by nerve fibre atrophy. Hence a cup:disc ratio greater than 0.6 is regarded as abnormal, raising the suspicion of glaucoma. Furthermore, 30 per cent of patients with glaucoma show asymmetry in the size of the physiological cup in the two eyes, whereas asymmetry occurs in only 5 per cent of normal individuals.

The margin of the optic disc is usually well defined, although the nasal boundary may be less distinct than that on the temporal side. In the majority of normal eyes there is no discontinuity between the margin of the disc and the adjacent retinal pigment epithelium and choroid. However, there are instances in which (because of oblique insertion of the optic nerve into the globe and consequent tilting of the disc) these layers fail to reach the disc margin. A gap in the retinal pigment epithelium reveals the underlying choroid; it may produce a dark juxtapapillary choroidal crescent (Fig. **6**), or may completely surround the optic disc to form a choroidal ring. When both the retinal pigment epithelium and choroid are deficient, a pale scleral crescent is the result (Fig. **7**). These two types of crescent most commonly arise on the temporal aspect of the optic disc; a scleral crescent is an invariable finding in *myopia* (*see* page 70). Alternatively, thickening of the retinal pigment epithelium may occur, resulting in a pigment crescent, most frequently related to the nasal aspect of the optic disc. None of the pigmentary changes are of pathological significance, but they have to be differentiated from those congenital and disease conditions showing peripapillary pigmentary abnormalities (e.g. *optic disc pit, see* page 26; *morning glory optic disc, see* page 31; *juxtapapillary choroiditis, see* page 108).

Retinal vessels

The central retinal artery enters the globe through the physiological cup. The vessel usually divides dichotomously within the cup and again on the surface of the disc, giving rise to four branches which supply the inferior and superior nasal and temporal quadrants of the fundus. Occasionally, the artery divides within the optic nerve head, so that two or four branches of the retinal artery emerge separately from within the physiological cup. The

5 A

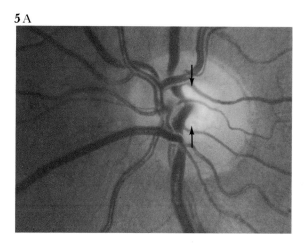

5 B

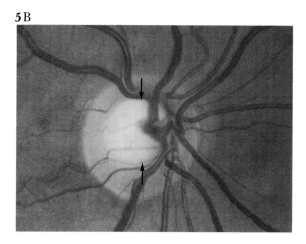

5   Normal variations in the size of the physiological cup (arrows). (**A**) cup:disc ratio, 0.3. (**B**) cup:disc ratio, 0.5.

arrangement of central retinal veins generally parallels that of the arteries, although the veins usually lie more temporally within the physiological cup. An anomalous distribution of the central retinal vessels in relation to the optic disc may be found in congenital abnormalities (e.g. *coloboma, morning glory optic disc, see* pages 21, 31) or acquired disorders (e.g. *glaucoma*).

Spontaneous pulsation of the central retinal vein occurs in nearly all normal eyes and is most clearly seen ophthalmoscopically at the physiological cup. Pulsation of the central retinal artery, on the other hand, is a manifestation of ocular or systemic disease; it may occur when intraocular pressure is very high (e.g. in *glaucoma*), or when pulse-pressure is elevated (e.g. in aortic incompetence).

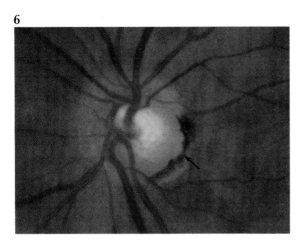

6 Choroidal crescent (arrow).

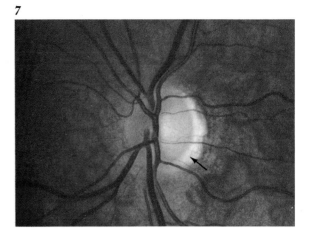

7 Juxtapapillary scleral crescent (arrow).

Cilioretinal arteries (*see* page 43) are present in 40 per cent of normal individuals. They are derived from the posterior ciliary circulation (*see* below) and usually emerge from the temporal aspect of the optic disc to supply a small portion of the retina; this may include capillaries in the macular region.

Retinal arterioles, arising from the central retinal arteries, are narrower than their accompanying venules (in the ratio 2:3). Thickening of the arterioles, as occurs in the generalized, age-related abnormality, arteriosclerosis, or in *hypertension* (*see* page 79), results in characteristic changes which can be seen ophthalmoscopically. These include a burnishing of the light reflex, known as 'copper-wiring'; further progression causes the arteriolar wall to become opaque and its contents obscured, giving the 'silver-wiring' appearance.

Morphology of the optic nerve head

Regional characteristics

The optic nerve head may be sub-divided anteroposteriorly into three regions: a surface layer, a prelaminar layer and the lamina cribrosa (Fig. **8**).

In the surface layer, non-myelinated nerve fibres originating from ganglion cells in the neural retina converge in the neural rim of the optic disc. In the prelaminar layer, these axons turn at right angles, perpendicular to the surface layer, and are directed posteriorly to

exit from the globe. Astroglial cells are present in the prelaminar layer and divide the nerve fibres into fascicles. In the third region these nerve-fibre bundles pass through fenestrations in the sieve-like lamina cribrosa (cribriform plate). The lamina cribrosa is situated in the scleral canal and is formed by connective tissue continuous with that of the surrounding sclera. Posterior to the lamina cribrosa, in the retrolaminar or retrobulbar portion of the optic nerve, axons of the nerves are myelinated.

Vascular supply

The vascular supply to the optic nerve head is derived from the central retinal and posterior ciliary circulations (Fig. **9**), both arising from the ophthalmic artery. There is a characteristic pattern of distribution in each of the three regions of the optic nerve head. Thus the surface layer is supplied by the central retinal circulation via capillaries arising on the optic disc from the main retinal vessels. If a cilioretinal artery is present, the surface layer may also receive capillaries derived from this vessel.

The deeper layers of the optic nerve head are supplied, directly or indirectly, from the posterior ciliary arteries. These originate from the ophthalmic artery and divide into about 20 short posterior ciliary arteries which enter the sclera around the optic nerve and are distributed to the choroid. Some of the short posterior ciliary arteries anastomose to form the circle of Zinn (often incomplete); this lies in the sclera, close to the optic nerve. From the circle of Zinn branches pass anteriorly to the choroid,

8

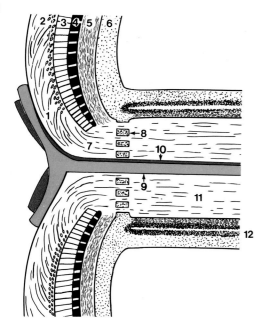

9

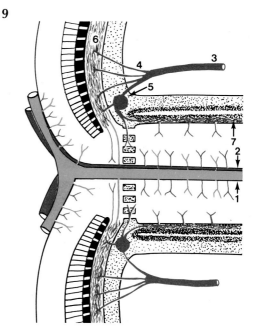

8   Section through the optic nerve head:
(1) surface layer of the optic disc;
(2) ganglion cell layer and retinal nerve fibre layer (non-myelinated);
(3) other layers of neural retina;
(4) retinal pigment epithelium;
(5) choroid;
(6) sclera;
(7) prelaminar layer;
(8) lamina cribrosa at the scleral canal (posterior limit of optic nerve head);
(9) central retinal vein;
(10) central retinal artery;
(11) optic nerve fibres (myelinated);
(12) dura, pia and arachnoid (with potential sub-arachnoid space); these meninges surround the retrobulbar portion of the optic nerve and are in continuity with the meninges of the brain.

9   Section through optic nerve head showing vascular supply:
(1) central retinal vein;
(2) central retinal artery;
(3) posterior ciliary artery;
(4) short posterior ciliary arteries;
(5) circle of Zinn;
(6) choroid;
(7) pial plexus.

centripetally to the lamina cribrosa and posteriorly to the pial network.

The prelaminar layer of the optic nerve head is supplied by centripetal branches from the choroidal circulation. In addition to branches from the circle of Zinn, the lamina cribrosa is supplied mainly by centripetal branches of the short posterior ciliary arteries. These branches are thought to be end arteries and their occlusion causes *ischaemic papillopathy* —as in, for example, *giant cell arteritis* (*see* pages 61, 62). The retrolaminar or retro-

bulbar portion of the optic nerve is supplied by small branches of the central retinal artery (running within the substance of the nerve) which pass centrifugally; it also receives centripetal branches from the surrounding pial plexus.

The venous drainage of the optic nerve head similarly involves the central retinal and choroidal circulations, the former being predominant. The central retinal vein is thought to drain all three regions of the optic nerve head but, in addition, small vessels in the

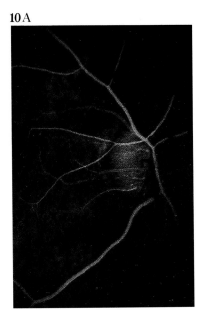 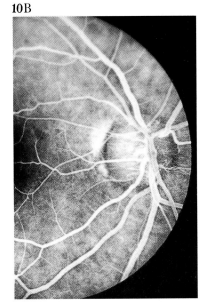 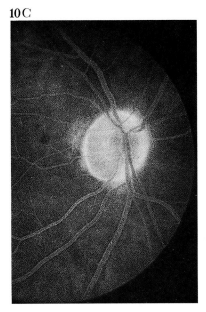

10   Fundus fluorescein angiogram of a normal optic disc.
(**A**) Early phase: the central retinal artery and disc capillaries begin to fill with dye. (**B**) Mid-phase: both the central retinal artery and vein are filled with dye. (**C**) Late phase: the central retinal vessels (now nearly devoid of dye) are silhouetted against the optic disc which stains late in the angiogram.

prelaminar layer may communicate with the choroidal circulation and then the vortex veins.

Fluorescein angiography

Fluorescein angiography can play an important role in the investigation of abnormalities involving the vascular supply to the optic disc and optic nerve head. In the normal individual the endothelium of capillaries in the optic nerve head is non-fenestrated, and therefore these vessels do not leak dye during the angiogram. In the late phase of the angiogram the optic disc often becomes stained with fluorescein, probably brought about by the retention of dye in the connective-tissue elements of the lamina cribrosa (Fig. **10**). This staining differs markedly from the leakage of dye observed in various disease conditions (e.g. *new vessels, see* page 54; *papilloedema, see* page 75).

Development—normal and abnormal

The primordia of the eye appear early in embryonic life but the development and differentiation of the components of this complex organ continue throughout the prenatal period, reaching completion after birth. Congenital disorders of the eye may therefore arise at all stages of intrauterine life. They represent anomalies in the developmental processes of growth, morphogenesis, differentiation and the remodelling which occurs, most notably, as the definitive ocular vasculature replaces the fetal system.

Optic primordia

The optic vesicles arise as paired, mushroom-shaped, hollow outgrowths from the primitive forebrain. Thus, in the 4th week after fertilization, they comprise a distal optic vesicle connected to the forebrain by a tubular optic stalk. Like the developing brain, they are composed of neuro-ectoderm. Failure of separation of the paired optic primordia, at a very early stage in their development, results in the rare, gross abnormality known as cyclopia, or single eye.

Normally, however, each optic vesicle grows laterally, becoming apposed to the overlying surface ectoderm. Once this relationship has been established, the surface ectoderm thickens to form a lens placode, which then invaginates to form a lens vesicle. Concomitantly, the optic vesicle becomes indented to form the optic cup, with the lens vesicle located at its mouth (Fig. **11**). The inverted inner layer of the optic cup undergoes rapid growth, deepening the invagination and bringing the future neural retina into relation with the outer layer of the cup (5–6 week embryo); the latter becomes the pigment layer of the retina. The most distal portion of the optic cup, curving anterior to the lens, will differentiate to form the pigment epithelium of the iris and its dilator and sphincter muscles (Fig. **12**).

Embryonic fissure

The invagination which transforms the optic vesicle into the optic cup also involves the optic stalk: thus, from the earliest stage in its formation until the 7th week of development, the cavity of the optic cup is in continuity with a groove—the embryonic fissure—which arises on the inferior aspect of the cup and runs along the inferior aspect of the tubular optic stalk (*see* Fig. **11**).

Mesenchyme lying within the fissure differentiates to form vascular tissue from which the hyaloid artery (later the central retinal artery) and the central retinal vein will be derived. During the 7th week of intrauterine life, as cells of the inner wall of the optic cup and stalk continue to proliferate, the lips of the embryonic fissure come together and begin to fuse. The process of fusion begins in the region of the future inferior peripheral retina; from this point it moves forwards towards the presumptive iris and pupillary region, and backwards to include the future optic disc and optic nerve. Any of these derivatives may be involved in failures of fusion which may occur anywhere along the length of the embryonic fissure and result in *colobomatous defects* (*see* page 21) and related disorders (e.g. *tilted disc syndrome, see* page 24). Such defects typically lie inferonasally within the eye, that is along the line of closure of the embryonic fissure (*see* Fig. **11**).

As a consequence of normal closure of the fissure, vascular mesenchyme (differentiating into the hyaloid artery) becomes incorporated into the substance of the optic stalk and exits from the optic cup at the site of the future optic disc. Part of the embryonic fissure proximal to the brain remains patent, and will do so throughout life; it marks the point of entry of the hyaloid artery and, later, the entry and exit of the central retinal vessels into the definitive optic nerve (*see* Fig. **9**).

Formation of the optic disc

The processes involved in the formation and differentiation of the optic disc and optic nerve head are, firstly, closure of the embryonic fissure (intimately related to cellular differentiation in the retina) and, secondly, modelling of the intraocular blood supply.

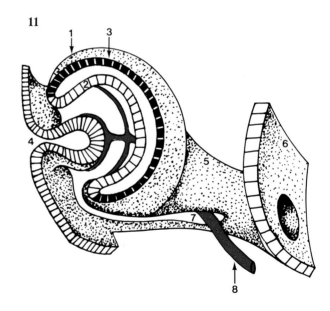

11 Optic primordia (5-week embryo). The optic vesicle has become invaginated to form a two-layered optic cup (1), in which neural (2) and pigment layers (3) of the future retina begin to differentiate. The lens (4) is formed from an invagination of the surface ectoderm. The optic cup and optic stalk (5), arising from the primitive forebrain (6), are grooved inferiorly by the embryonic fissure (7) which contains the hyaloid artery (8).

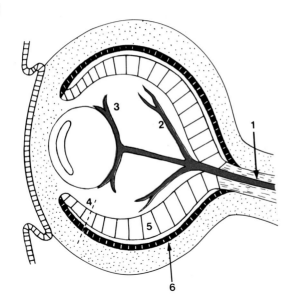

The hyaloid artery (1) lies within the substance of the optic nerve and enters the globe at the optic disc. One group of its branch vessels (vasa hyaloidia propria (2)) supplies the primary vitreous; another group is associated with the posterior surface of the lens (posterior tunica vasculosa lentis (3)). That portion of the two-layered optic cup lying anterior to the lens will form the iris (4); posteriorly it differentiates ito neural retina (5) and retinal pigment epithelium (6).

Cellular differentiation in the retina begins 5–6 weeks after conception, when pigment granules first accumulate in cells in the outer layer of the optic cup. The future neural retina, derived from the inner layer of the optic cup, also begins to take form, although it is not until the 6th month of development that all the layers of the adult retina can be recognized. However, as early as the 7th week, nerve processes arising from retinal ganglion cells grow backwards and converge radially at the junction between the optic cup and optic stalk. Here they turn at right angles out of the optic cup, to run in the substance of the optic stalk towards the brain, thereby establishing intra- and extraocular portions of the optic nerve. Absence or a reduction in the number of nerve fibres in the optic nerve gives rise to the conditions known as *aplasia* and *hypoplasia*, respectively (*see* page 28); *congenital optic atrophy* (*see* page 67) represents a secondary degeneration of optic nerve fibres taking place after birth.

Even before the arrival and convergence of the nerve processes, the position of the presumptive optic disc is marked by the presence of an elevation, the primitive epithelial papilla, located at the junction between optic cup and optic stalk. Abnormal differentiation of neural and pigment epithelial cells in this region is thought to be responsible for the formation of *congenital optic disc pits* (*see* page 26). After closure of the embryonic fissure the hyaloid artery and, later, the definitive retinal vessels pass within the substance of the optic nerve to enter or exit from the globe through the central region of the optic disc. In addition, as the nerve processes arising from retinal ganglion cells penetrate the epithelial papilla, cells of the papilla—isolated superficially and centrally on the surface of the developing optic disc—form a cone-shaped mass called Bergmeister's papilla. The cells of this papilla form a glial and fibrous network which supports the hyaloid artery as it enters the globe and runs forwards towards the posterior aspect of the lens (Fig. **13**).

Neuro-ectodermal cells, invaginated into the optic stalk during closure of the embryonic fissure, give rise to the neuroglial supporting cells of the optic nerve. Invading mesenchymal cells (together with an increasing number of nerve processes passing from the retina towards the brain) also contribute in the transformation of the tubular optic stalk into the solid structure of the optic nerve. An excess of non-neural, supporting elements in the optic nerve head causes *megalopapilla*, or enlargement of the optic disc (*see* page 30).

While differentiation of structures derived from primitive neuro-ectoderm is taking place, mesoderm surrounding the optic cup and stalk becomes condensed and differentiates to form the sclera anteriorly. Posterior to the globe of the eye, mesoderm forms the dura, arachnoid and pia which envelop the extraocular portion of the optic nerve as well as the brain (*see* Fig. **8**).

Differentiation within the optic nerve involves the establishment of longitudinal septa formed

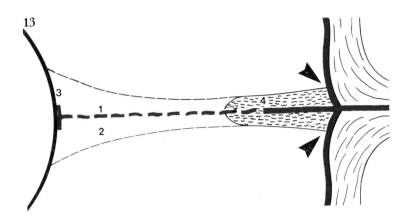

13 The eye during late fetal life. The intra-ocular portion of the hyaloid artery (1) regresses; the vessel is partially sheathed by remnants of the primary vitreous (2) which is attached to the posterior surface of the lens (3). Regression of Bergmeister's papilla (4) determines the degree of physiological cupping of the optic disc (arrows).

by glial cells. In the posterior layer of the optic nerve head these tissues are augmented by capillary and connective-tissue mesenchyme, originating from the sclera, to form the sieve-like lamina cribrosa. Two congenital abnormalities are thought to be associated with defective development of the sclera and lamina cribrosa. Enlargement of the scleral foramen and posterior displacement of the lamina cribrosa, with prolapse of the optic nerve head, may be responsible for the *morning glory disc anomaly* (*see* page 31). Conversely, a reduction in the area of the lamina cribrosa is believed to be the factor primarily responsible for inhibition of axonal flow and accumulation of material in the optic nerve head, to produce *optic disc drusen* (*see* page 81).

Myelination of optic nerve fibres, effected by oligodendroglia cells, is initiated within the central nervous system during the 6th month of fetal life. The process of myelination in the optic nerve extends peripherally to reach the lamina cribrosa around the time of birth, where it normally halts. *Atypical myelination* in the optic disc and retina may continue postnatally, however, presumably brought about by the presence of oligodendrocytes anterior to the cribriform plate (*see* page 34).

Many of the congenital abnormalities arising during the formation and organization of the optic nerve head are non-progressive. On the other hand, what is believed to be an inherited form of *axial myopia* involves growth discrepancies in the eye which, in its most serious manifestation, may progress until late in adult life (*see* page 70). *Hypermetropia*, similarly, is a congenital abnormality; in this condition the eye is smaller than normal (*see* page 84).

Vascular elements associated with the optic disc

The hyaloid vessels supply and drain the interior of the eye during the period of its most active growth and differentiation. The intra-ocular portion of the hyaloid system normally atrophies during the latter part of fetal life, when organization of the eye is almost complete. However, those portions of the vessels that remain within the substance of the optic nerve persist, having already become established as the definitive central retinal artery and central retinal vein.

The hyaloid artery, derived from the internal carotid via its ophthalmic branch, enters the embryonic fissure in about the 4th week (*see* Fig. **11**) and runs forwards within the optic cup to form two groups of vessels. One group supplies the vascular and fibrous syncytium of the primary vitreous (vasa hyaloidia propria) and the other group ramifies over the posterior surface of the lens (posterior tunica vasculosa lentis) (*see* Fig. **12**). Connections are also established, anterior to the lens, between the hyaloid system and the future vessels of the iris.

The hyaloid system reaches the height of its development in the 3rd month of intrauterine life: the first stages of its subsequent regression are correlated with the formation of the secondary, definitive vitreous. The latter, which progressively supplants the vascular primary vitreous, is a fibrous, gelatinous, avascular derivative of the retina. The primary vitreous becomes restricted to a strand of tissue traversing the secondary vitreous, with a central canal (Cloquet's canal) containing the hyaloid artery and, subsequently, its arterial remnants.

The tissues of the primary vitreous are contiguous with the glial and fibrous tissue of Bergmeister's papilla which, at the height of its development in the 6th month, ensheaths the hyaloid artery in the first one-third of its course through the secondary vitreous (*see* Fig. **13**). The intraocular portion of the hyaloid artery atrophies during the last few weeks of gestation, following regression of the tunica vasculosa lentis. Bergmeister's papilla also atrophies during the latter part of the fetal period, the degree to which it regresses determining the amount of physiological cupping in the definitive optic disc (*see* Fig. **13**). A spectrum of congenital abnormalities is represented by *persistence of the hyaloid artery*, and/or *Bergmeister's papilla*, and/or the *primary vitreous* (*see* pages 36–41).

Precursors of the definitive retinal circulation appear during the 4th month, when capillaries are established in the inner layers of the retina. From this time onwards, that portion of the hyaloid artery that lies within the optic nerve and supplies the developing and definitive retina should be known as the central retinal artery. The dynamics of blood flow within the primitive retinal capillary network determine the definitive vascular pattern. Upper and lower temporal and nasal retinal arteries differentiate as major channels, with retinal venous vessels developing roughly in parallel. The central retinal vein develops within the optic nerve from vascular elements associated with the hyaloid artery (3rd month). Congenital anomalies of the retinal vessels are represented by the development of aberrant vascular channels (e.g. *prepapillary loops*, *see* page 38; *retinal macrovessels*, *see* page 46; *racemose haemangioma*, *see* page 47). Among other vascular anomalies arising during prenatal life, *situs inversus* (*see* page 42) rarely appears as an isolated phenomenon but is almost exclusively associated with other abnormalities. *Cilioretinal vessels* (*see* page 43) are thought to represent a normal variation of the optic disc vasculature.

Other congenital abnormalities affecting the optic disc include the hamartomas and some neoplasms. *Hamartomas* are tumour-like malformations arising during the process of tissue differentiation (*see* page 87), for example *astrocytic hamartoma* (*see* page 87). Congenital tumours that may affect the optic disc include *melanocytoma* (*see* page 85) and the highly malignant *retinoblastoma* (*see* page 98).

2: Non-Progressive Congenital Abnormalities

Most congenital abnormalities of the optic disc are non-progressive and untreatable. Accurate diagnosis is essential, however, to distinguish these conditions from other congenital and acquired ocular disorders which affect vision progressively and may be amenable to treatment. In addition, some non-progressive congenital anomalies of the optic disc are associated with systemic abnormalities which may have serious implications for the patient if not diagnosed.

Coloboma

Colobomas arise early in the development of the eye and are caused by failure of fusion of the embryonic fissure (*see* page 17). They are defects that usually lie inferiorly and may affect one, or more than one, of the following structures: optic disc, retina, choroid, inferior iris and lens. Colobomas commonly occur bilaterally; most cases arise sporadically, or are inherited in an autosomal dominant pattern.

There are three types of coloboma that occur in association with the optic disc and fundus. The first is a coloboma of the optic nerve head; this is an extremely rare condition. The second and most common form is retinochoroidal coloboma which affects the neural retina, retinal pigment epithelium and choroid. The third type of coloboma, known as the tilted disc syndrome, probably also involves incomplete closure of the embryonic fissure; it is described as a separate entity (*see* page 24).

(i) Isolated coloboma of the optic nerve head

Ophthalmoscopy
(Fig. **14**)

1. The optic disc is enlarged and may be partially or almost totally excavated. The deepest part of the coloboma is usually situated inferiorly, where the margin of the optic disc may lose its integrity.
2. The coloboma is glistening white in colour, sometimes tinged with grey on its surface.
3. Characteristically, an increased number of retinal blood vessels cross the border of the coloboma; they represent branches of the central retinal vessels which have divided on the surface of the enlarged optic disc before reaching the retina.
4. Peripapillary pigmentary changes (hyper- or hypopigmentation) are common.

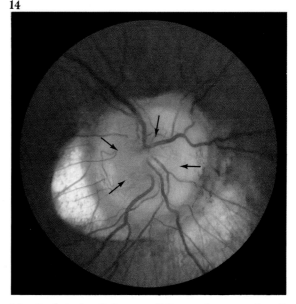

14 Isolated coloboma of the optic nerve head (arrows) showing enlarged disc with numerous vessels crossing its border; the disc margin is indistinct. There are two areas of juxtapapillary hypopigmentation and patches of pigment clumping.

Supplementary findings

Visual acuity is variably affected and any reduction is related, not to the size of the lesion as seen ophthalmoscopically, but to the extent of neural involvement. Colour vision may also be affected.

Visual field abnormalities are variable, often showing a general constriction and centro-caecal defect, or enlargement of the blind spot with arcuate or ring scotomas. These defects are generally non-progressive, except when an associated retinal detachment develops.

Serous retinal detachments occur quite commonly; they are generally non-rhegmatogenous (i.e. without holes or tears) and usually develop in early adult life. When they occur, the prognosis for retention of visual acuity is poor. The source of the sub-retinal fluid associated with the detachment is unknown.

Associated ocular features include posterior lenticonus, congenital optic disc pit, cyst of the optic nerve sheath, hyaloid artery remnants, posterior embryotoxin and myopia. Strabismus is an important presenting sign in children.

Associated systemic features

These include trans-sphenoidal encephalocoele, as well as cardiac defects, ear dysplasias and facial nerve palsy.

Differential diagnosis

See under (ii) below.

(ii) Retinochoroidal coloboma

Ophthalmoscopy
(Figs. **15**, **16**)

1. There is a white, well-defined, usually circular area located in the inferonasal fundus; it may be contiguous with a coloboma of the optic disc, or may occur independently.
2. The retinal border of the lesion is commonly pigmented.

15
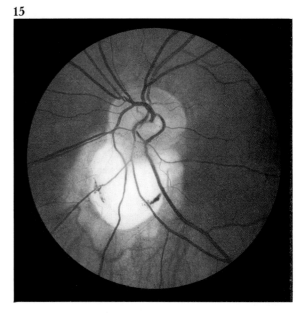

16
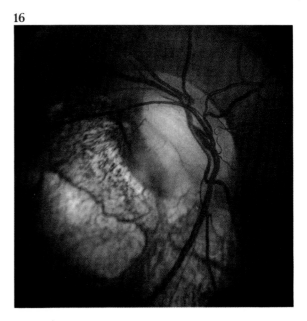

15 Retinochoroidal coloboma extending infero-nasally from the optic disc.

16 Retinochoroidal coloboma contiguous with coloboma of the optic disc.

Supplementary findings

Effects on visual acuity, colour vision and visual field defects are similar to those described for (i) above. Retinal detachments may occur, but are often rhegmatogenous (i.e. due to a tear or hole in the retina, cf. (i) above); such detachments may be progressive, owing to subretinal neovascularization or haemorrhage.

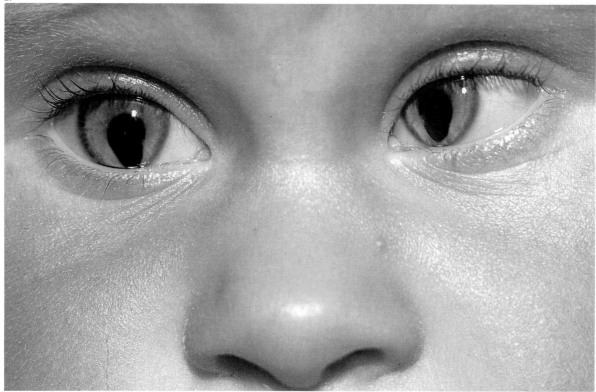

17 Bilateral coloboma of the iris.

As might be expected, associated ocular features include defects that involve failure of fusion of the most anterior extremities of the embryonic fissure, for example coloboma of the iris (Fig. **17**) or aniridia. Other related abnormalities include staphyloma of the sclera, persistent hyperplastic primary vitreous, microphthalmia, microcornea, cataract and posterior embryotoxin. Strabismus may again be a presenting feature, particularly if the defect is unilateral; the patient may be either myopic or hypermetropic.

Associated systemic features

Although colobomas may occur as isolated defects, systemic abnormalities associated with retinochoroidal colobomas are numerous and may be severe; they involve the cardiovascular, central nervous and musculoskeletal systems, the gastrointestinal and genitourinary tracts, and the nasopharynx and the ears.

Differential diagnosis

(Applicable to both (i) and (ii) above.)
Colobomas should be differentiated from other abnormalities in which the optic disc is:

1. Excavated, and
2. Apparently enlarged.
3. There is peripapillary pigmentary change.

Tilted disc syndrome
(Nasal fundus ectasia syndrome; Fuchs' coloboma; Dysversion of the optic disc)

Tilting of the optic disc can occur in any direction, although in this condition the disc is usually inclined inferiorly or inferonasally. It presents in association with a number of other anomalies (namely: inferior nasal crescent, situs inversus of the retinal vessels, fundus ectasia, myopia, astigmatism, visual field defects) all or some of which, in combination, constitute the tilted disc syndrome.

The morphological features of this fairly common congenital abnormality are comparatively insignificant. However, the syndrome is important clinically since it may cause bitemporal visual field loss and must therefore be distinguished from serious disorders of the central nervous system, such as pituitary tumour, which involve the optic chiasma and similarly affect the visual field.

The condition is thought to be a form of coloboma brought about by defective closure of the embryonic fissure (*see* page 17) which, in this instance, causes the optic nerve to enter the globe of the eye at an unusual angle. This results in tilting of the optic nerve head and dysversion (change in orientation) of the physiological optic cup, so that the central axis of the cup deviates from the temporal towards the nasal side and the retinal vessels are displaced (situs inversus). The location of other associated abnormalities in the inferior fundus supports the thesis that the defect arises at the site of the embryonic fissure.

The syndrome affects 1–2 per cent of the population and 75 per cent of cases occur bilaterally. It has been reported as a familial trait, but no inheritance pattern has been defined.

Ophthalmoscopy
(Figs. **18**, **19**)

1. The optic disc is tilted, usually superiorly–inferiorly and with its vertical axis directed obliquely so that the upper temporal portion of the disc lies anterior to its lower margin (an appearance that may be mistaken for papilloedema, *see* page 75).
2. Associated with the lower margin of the disc there is usually a crescent of exposed choroid or sclera. This, in turn, is often related to an area of hypopigmentation (ectasia) affecting the inferonasal portion of the retina.
3. Situs inversus is present in about 80 per cent of eyes with a tilted disc. In this condition (brought about by dysversion of the optic cup) the temporal retinal vessels first turn nasally as they emerge from the optic disc, before curving temporally towards the macula.

Supplementary findings

Visual acuity is normal in 25 per cent of cases and minimally decreased in the remainder; the patient is usually unaware of any decrement. The greater the tilt or displacement of the disc, the lower the visual acuity and the more severe any associated astigmatism and/or myopia. Unilateral cases predispose to amblyopia and strabismus.

It has been suggested that decreased visual acuity is secondary to the Stiles–Crawford effect. This presupposes that not only the optic disc but also part of the retina lies obliquely to the visual axis, so that light strikes the lateral aspect of the photoreceptors rather than their proximal ends.

There is a superior temporal or bitemporal visual field loss which is non-progressive and correlates well with the defective area of the disc. This visual field deficit can be distinguished from those brought about by pressure on the optic chiasma since, in the former, the defect crosses the vertical meridian so that the nasal sector is also involved (Fig. **20**).

Fundus fluorescein angiography can be used to distinguish between cases of the tilted disc syndrome and papilloedema (*see* page 75).

Associated systemic features

None known.

Differential diagnosis

Cases of tilted disc should be differentiated from other abnormalities in which the optic disc appears hyperaemic and swollen.

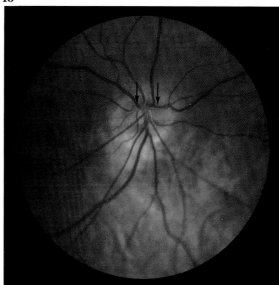

18 Inferiorly tilted optic disc. The superior central retinal vessels emerge from beneath the upper rim (arrows) of the disc.

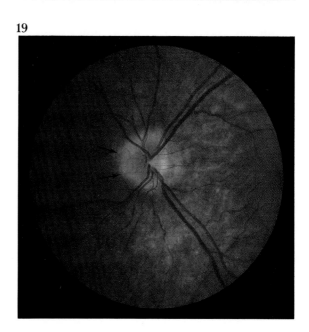

19 Lateral tilting of left optic disc. In this less typical condition, the nasal margin of the disc (arrows) is elevated and indistinct.

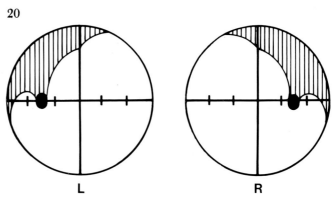

20 Bitemporal hemianopia associated with tilted discs. The defect crosses the vertical meridian to involve the nasal sector in each eye.

Optic disc pit

A congenital optic disc pit is thought to represent an abnormality arising early in the development of the presumptive optic disc (epithelial papilla), before differentiation of the neural retina and optic nerve head (*see* page 18).

The abnormality occurs quite commonly. It consists of a depression in the optic disc, often darker in appearance than the disc itself. The lesion is frequently situated in the temporal region of the optic disc and does not affect the disc margin (cf. coloboma, *see* page 21). Usually only one eye is affected (85 per cent of cases); there is no known hereditary pattern.

Ophthalmoscopy
(Figs. **21**, **22**)

1. The pit takes the form of a round or oval depression in the optic disc and is often pigmented.
2. The margin of the optic disc is complete and is not interrupted by the presence of the pit; the physiological optic cup also remains distinct.
3. The base of the pit may be seen to pulsate, these pulsations being transmitted either from underlying blood vessels, or from the sub-arachnoid space.
4. The pits vary in size, occupying from one-quarter to half of the disc diameter, with a depth ranging between 0.5 dioptre and 20–25 dioptre (mean c. 5 dioptre): the optic disc in which a congenital pit occurs is larger than the disc in the contralateral, unaffected eye.
5. There is usually only one pit per optic disc, although two or three occasionally occur.
6. Peripapillary chorioretinal atrophy, with changes in the pigment epithelium, are seen in almost all of those cases where the pit is situated peripherally, near to the margin of the optic disc.

Two vascular variants are associated with the congenital optic pit:

1. In 60 per cent of cases a cilioretinal artery can be identified, arising from the periphery of the pit (cf. a 40 per cent occurrence in normal eyes; *see* page 43).
2. In other instances, retinal vessels are seen to cross the optic pit, either running superficially or dipping below its surface. (The latter observation raises the question of whether the frequency of an associated cilioretinal artery has been over-estimated

21

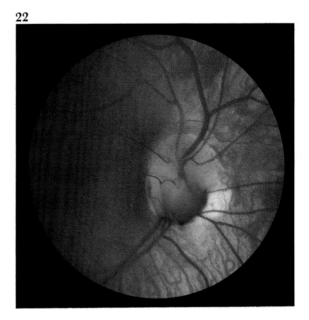

21 An optic disc pit. The pit (arrow) is olive grey and situated in the temporal area; there is a crescent of pigmentation on the adjacent disc margin.

22 An optic disc pit involves the inferior area of the disc but not its margin. The lower central retinal vessels emerge from the base of the pit.

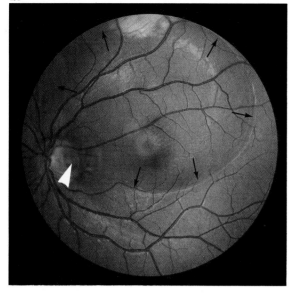

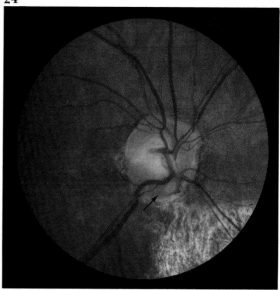

23 A large serous retinal detachment is associated with an optic disc pit (triangle). The detachment (arrows) extends from the temporal margin of the optic disc, which additionally shows pigmentary change.

    —a vessel emerging at the periphery of the defect possibly representing the terminal portion of a retinal artery.)
3. Another ophthalmoscopic finding is that of a serous retinal detachment (Fig. **23**) which develops in 30 per cent of cases. This complication, generally related to larger pits in the temporal region of the disc, extends from the disc margin. The detachment is characterized by the presence of small, yellow deposits, lying on the posterior surface of the detached portion of the retina and believed to represent aggregates of pigment-laden macrophages. These detachments typically resolve spontaneously and the yellow deposits disappear, although the cycle may be repeated. If the detachment persists, a secondary degenerative macular hole may develop.

Supplementary findings

Visual acuity is usually good and the condition is most often discovered in the course of a routine eye examination.

Vision may be affected, however, by the development of a serous retinal detachment, most commonly presenting during the fourth decade (although this complication has been reported in the first and ninth decades of life).

24 An optic disc pit in an inferior position on the disc (arrow) is associated with a retinochoroidal coloboma.

Such patients suffer from distortion of the vision, but only 5 per cent have a visual acuity of less than 6/36. The mechanism of production of the subretinal fluid associated with a serous detachment is controversial. Some consider that it originates from cerebrospinal fluid which leaks into the subretinal space; others suggest that it derives from the vitreous, entering via a macular hole; a third view is that seepage from blood vessels at the base of the pit is the source.

Numerous visual field abnormalities are reported, usually extending from the optic disc: the most common are arcuate (40 per cent) or centrocaecal defects although others, such as nasal or temporal defects, may occur.

Other related ocular anomalies include persistent hyaloid artery, retinochoroidal coloboma (Fig. **24**) and iris coloboma.

Associated systemic features

There are generally none, although—as in other instances of optic disc dysplasia—a basal encephalocoele of the skull may occur.

Differential diagnosis

Optic disc pits need to be differentiated from other abnormalities in which the optic disc appears: 1. Excavated. 2. Enlarged. 3. There is peripapillary pigmentary change.

Aplasia and hypoplasia

Absence or a reduction in the number of nerve fibres in the optic nerve gives rise to the conditions known as aplasia and hypoplasia, respectively. Aplasia is seldom seen since it is often linked with anencephaly and other major cranial maldevelopments, incompatible with life.

Hypoplasia of the optic disc results from failure of development of the ganglion cell layer in the neural retina (*see* page 18). Whether this represents the primary defect, or whether it arises secondary to a congenital lesion in the cerebral hemispheres with retrograde degeneration of the optic nerve fibres, remains to be established.

In hypoplasia the optic disc is reduced in size and those nerve fibres that remain are concentrated centrally, forming a contracted disc, encircled by aberrant tissue. The latter often forms an inner and outer annulus of pigment with the outer ring of pigment overlying the junction between the lamina cribrosa and sclera (i.e. corresponding to the true outer margin of a normal optic disc).

The condition occurs unilaterally or bilaterally, with equal frequency. Although it usually arises sporadically, familial cases have been described. Iatrogenic correlations have also been reported. For example, hypoplasia of the optic disc is more common in the children of mothers with epilepsy, who used anticonvulsant drugs during pregnancy, and in the children of mothers who took quinine or LSD; the children of diabetic mothers may also be affected.

Ophthalmoscopy

There are three cardinal signs (Figs. **25**, **26**):

1. The optic nerve head is small and the disc may be reduced to one-third of its normal size.
2. A 'double ring sign' can be identified around the periphery of the hypoplastic disc; it consists of two concentric rings of pigment with an intervening cuff of paler tissue; the disc itself may be mottled with pigment.
3. The retinal vessels are usually of normal calibre, but exit and enter centrally from the shrunken disc (cf. their slightly eccentric, nasal position in the normal disc).

In addition, the foveal reflex may be absent.

Supplementary findings

The visual acuity is variable. It may be normal, but more commonly is reduced from the time of birth; this reduction is non-progressive. If visual acuity is low, the pupil may react poorly to light. Colour vision may also be affected.

Visual field defects show many patterns, including bitemporal and binasal hemianopias (the former mimicking the effect of a pituitary tumour compressing the optic chiasma).

Associated ocular features include nystagmus, strabismus, retinochoroidal coloboma, microphthalmia, microcornea, blepharoptosis and palsies of the 3rd, 4th and 6th cranial nerves.

Associated systemic features

There are a considerable number of related systemic abnormalities, many of them affecting mid-line cranial and cerebral structures, with severe cases involving anencephaly or hydrocephaly. These are particularly likely to arise in patients with bilateral optic disc hypoplasia.

In De Morsier's syndrome (septo-optic dysplasia) absence of the septum pellucidum results in a single anterior cerebral vesicle (as demonstrated by means of computerized tomography). In addition, because of pituitary hypoplasia, neonates are prone to hypoglycaemic seizures; growth hormone deficiency results in dwarfism.

Other systemic abnormalities include various forms of craniofacial maldevelopment, also deafness and congenital heart disease. Cases with bilateral optic disc hypoplasia are also prone to develop congenital tumours in the region of the optic chiasma (e.g. craniopharyngioma, optic nerve glioma).

Differential diagnosis

Hypoplasia should be differentiated from other conditions in which the optic disc is:

1. Small; and
2. There is associated peripapillary pigmentary change.

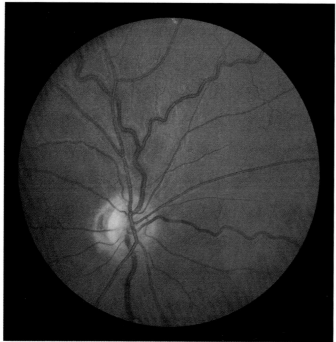

25 Hypoplasia. The optic disc is reduced in size and surrounded by a pale annulus. Retinal vessels are of normal calibre but emerge centrally from the optic disc.

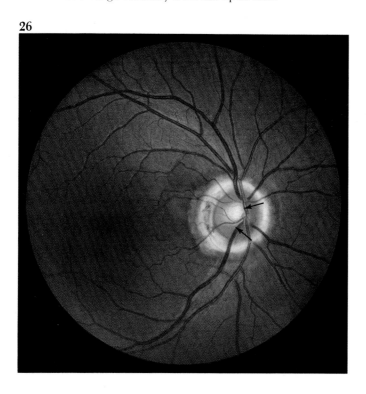

26 'Double ring sign' in hypoplasia of the optic disc. In this case the retinal vessels emerge from the normal, slightly nasal position (arrows) on the disc.

Megalopapilla

27 A

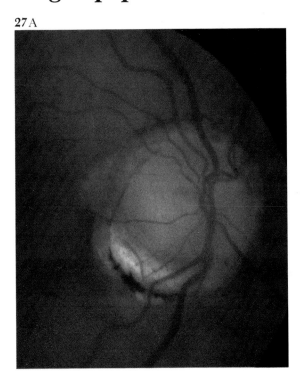

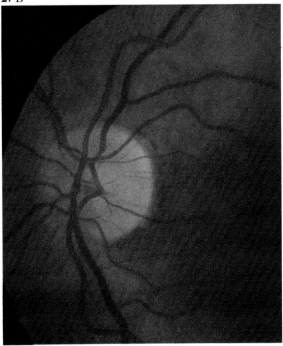

3. Some pigmentary changes may present in the peripapillary region.

27 (A) Megalopapilla, with pigmentary changes visible at the inferior margin of the disc. (**B**) Optic disc of normal size, in the fellow eye.

Megalopapilla reflects abnormal development of the optic nerve head brought about by an increase, either of neural supporting tissue, or of the amount of mesodermal tissue infiltrating the nerve (*see* page 18).

In this rare congenital abnormality the optic disc is enlarged—it may be up to double the normal size—but its appearance is otherwise mainly unchanged. The condition usually occurs unilaterally, although both eyes are occasionally affected. There is no known inheritance pattern.

Ophthalmoscopy
(Fig. **27**)

1. The optic disc is enlarged, but is otherwise normal in appearance.
2. Because of the enlargement of the optic disc, the retinal blood vessels may appear narrowed; however, comparison with vessels in the unaffected fellow eye will show them to be of normal calibre.

Supplementary findings

Visual acuity is generally normal, but if slightly reduced may cause a child to present with strabismus. Refraction is usually emmetropic, although myopia sometimes occurs. The visual field may show an enlarged blind spot.

Associated systemic features

These are potentially severe and all relate to mid-line defects in the development of the skull and face: they include spheno-ethmoidal encephalocoele, basal encephalocoele and cleft palate. Radiological investigation is therefore indicated for patients with megalopapilla. The optic foramen, although slightly enlarged, remains within the normal range (cf. glioma, *see* page 95).

Differential diagnosis

Megalopapilla has to be distinguished from other abnormal conditions associated with:

1. An enlarged optic disc; and
2. Peripapillary pigmentary change.

Morning glory optic disc

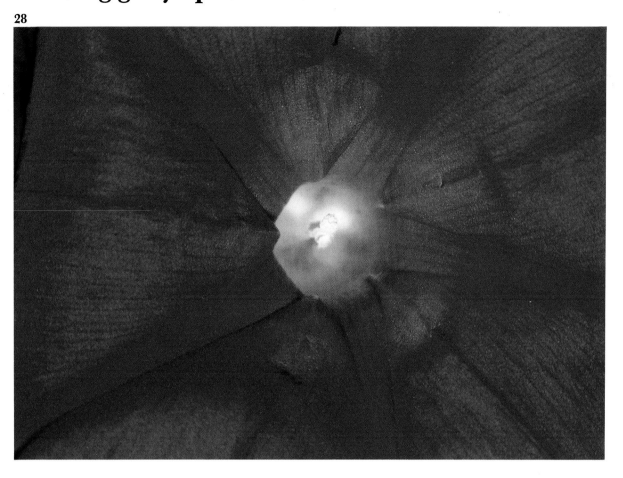

28 Morning glory.

In this rare developmental anomaly, the physiological optic cup is replaced by a central, funnel-shaped depression in the disc, having a core of white tissue; there is also a pigmented juxtapapillary annulus. The name of the condition derives from its shape and the concentric arrangement of the variously coloured tissues of the disc and annulus, which bear a resemblance to the trumpet-shaped flower, morning glory (Fig. **28**).

There are several theories concerning the aetiology of the disorder. The first is that morning glory optic disc is a colobomatous defect, although the depression is situated centrally, whereas disorders affecting abnormal closure of the embryonic fissure usually arise inferiorly in relation to the optic disc. A more attractive thesis is that the depression in the disc is brought about by prolapse of the optic nerve head and posterior displacement of the lamina cribrosa, due to an enlarged scleral foramen (features seen in histological studies) (*see* page 19). A third proposal is based upon an observed similarity between the white core of tissue in the morning glory disc, and the more anteriorly placed, pale remnants identified as persistent hyperplastic primary vitreous (*see* page 40); it is suggested that the two conditions represent the extremes of what is fundamentally a continuum of the same disorder.

Morning glory optic disc is nearly always a unilateral defect; it occurs more commonly in the right eye, and in females rather than males (in the ratio 2:1). It is usually associated with poor visual acuity. There is no known hereditary pattern.

Ophthalmoscopy

There are three cardinal signs (Figs. **29**, **30**):

1. The optic disc appears enlarged and contains a deep, conical depression with white tissue at its base (cf. persistent hyperplastic primary vitreous, *see* page 40). The neural rim of the optic disc may be pink and normal in appearance.
2. A raised annulus surrounds the optic disc; it contains a variable amount of pigment and may present as a grey or black 'halo' to the disc, probably containing atrophic material of chorioretinal origin.
3. The retinal blood vessels loop over the edge of the disc in a radial fashion, like the spokes of a wheel; the origin and early branching of the arteries is frequently obscured by the white tissue in the central cone. Vessels tend to be sheathed near to the disc.

An additional feature which may be seen on ophthalmoscopy is a serous retinal detachment, extending peripherally from the disc. The detachment may fluctuate and resolve spontaneously.

Supplementary findings

Visual acuity is often poor from birth and the patient may present with strabismus. In severe cases an afferent pupillary reflex may be observed. The visual field may contain a centrocaecal scotoma.

Associated ocular features include remnants of the hyaloid artery, preretinal gliosis, myopia and eyelid abnormalities. On radiological examination the optic foramen is found to be of normal size, suggesting that the optic nerve is of normal calibre, even though the optic disc appears enlarged.

Associated systemic features

As with other dysplasias of the optic nerve head, mid-line defects of the skull and face may occur: they include basal encephalocoele, defective or absent floor of the sella turcica and ocular hypertelorism.

Differential diagnosis

Morning glory optic disc has to be differentiated from other abnormalities in which the disc appears:

1. Excavated;
2. Enlarged; and
3. There is peripapillary pigmentary change.

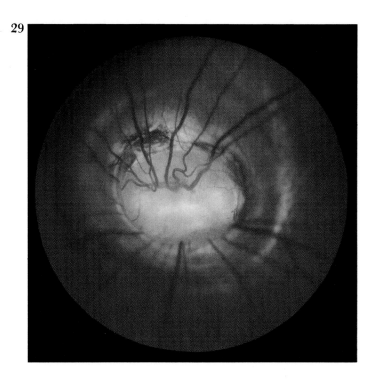

29 Morning glory optic disc with pale central core and surrounding raised annulus. The central retinal vessels radiate over the rim of the hollow cone.

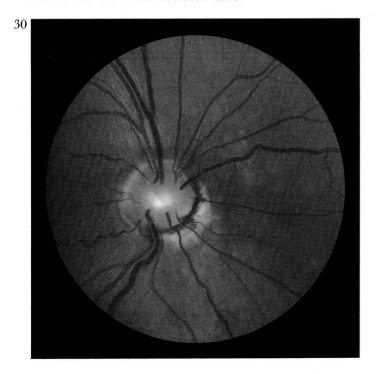

30 Morning glory optic disc; a less severe example.

Myelinated nerve fibres

This condition affects the myelination of nerve fibres in the optic disc and retina. It is a fairly common, usually asymptomatic anomaly found in about 1 per cent of the population. It is not present at birth, but appears postnatally (*see* page 19). There is no known hereditary pattern.

Ophthalmoscopy
(Figs **31–33**)

1. Myelinated nerve fibres form a white, highly reflective lesion which has feathery margins; dark 'slits' within the lesion represent normal, unmyelinated fibres.
2. Located in the superficial retina, the myelin sheaths partially obscure underlying structures such as blood vessels, the course and calibre of which is not affected.
3. The area of myelination may be large or small; it usually extends from the optic disc and often shows a fan-like distribution corresponding with that of the retinal nerve fibres; isolated patches of myelin occur in the peripheral retina, but infrequently.

Supplementary findings

Myelinated nerve fibres are almost always asymptomatic and an incidental finding during routine fundus examination. A small visual field defect may be identified on detailed testing; it is non-progressive and may take the form of an enlarged blind spot or arcuate defect, coincident with the distribution of afferent nerve fibres. Generally the affected eye is otherwise normal; rarely there may be associated ocular disorders such as myopia, amblyopia or strabismus and—even more rarely—coloboma, polycoria or keratoconus. If any of these conditions is present there may also be nystagmus.

Associated systemic features

Malformations of the skull, such as oxycephaly, are found very occasionally. Myelinated nerve fibres have also been reported in association with neurofibromatosis (*see under* astrocytic hamartoma, page 87).

Differential diagnosis

Myelinated nerve fibres of the optic disc have to be differentiated from those disc abnormalities that show:

1. An apparently enlarged disc.
2. A pale, swollen disc.

Myelinated nerve fibres in the peripheral retina have to be distinguished from cotton-wool spots caused by retinal ischaemia (e.g., as in diabetes and hypertension; *see* pages 55, 79).

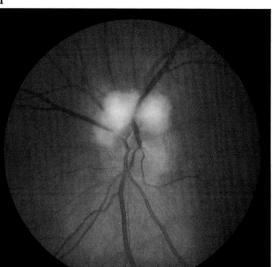

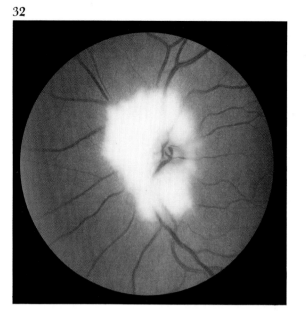

31 White myelinated nerve fibres extend from the optic disc into the adjacent retina, partially obscuring the disc margin and major vessels.

32 Myelination totally involving the optic disc; its extension into the surrounding retina shows the feathery margin typical of the lesion. The patient was asymptomatic.

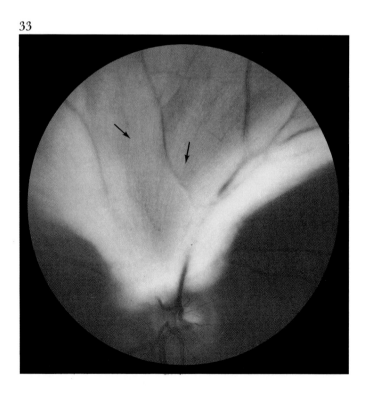

33 Fan-like pattern of myelination, following the distribution of the retinal nerve fibres. The dark slits (arrows) represent normal, non-myelinated fibres.

3: Vascular Abnormalities

Congenital vascular anomalies

Remnants of the fetal vascular tree and vitreous

Although the intraocular portion of the hyaloid artery normally regresses during late fetal life, all or part of the vessel may persist postnatally, as may its associated tissues. The latter comprise the glial and fibrous supporting elements of Bergmeister's papilla on the optic disc, and cells of the primary vitreous more anteriorly. Thus remnants of structures functional in the fetal eye may persist, either singly or in combination, and present as a range of congenital abnormalities which reflect their close developmental and morphological relationships. In addition, vascular loops that arise in Bergmeister's papilla may present as aberrant branches of the definitive retinal vessels, extending forwards from the optic disc.

Persistent hyaloid artery

Remnants of the hyaloid artery (*see* page 19) can be identified in 95 per cent of premature infants but in less than 5 per cent of infants at full term; their prevalence in adults is uncertain. They usually occur unilaterally. Remnants of the vessel extend forwards from the optic disc towards the lens.

Ophthalmoscopy

1. A persistent hyaloid artery generally presents as a bloodless, transparent, threadlike remnant extending forwards from the optic disc (Fig. **34**).
2. Occasionally the portion nearest to the optic disc contains blood.
3. Anteriorly the artery may retain its attachment to the posterior capsule of the lens. The point of attachment typically lies inferonasally to the visual axis and forms a small opacity, known as Mittendorf's dot (Fig. **35**). The latter may be the only remnant found in adults on ophthalmoscopic or slit-lamp examination.

Supplementary findings

A persistent hyaloid artery is usually asymptomatic. However, if the lumen of the vessel remains patent, vitreous haemorrhage may occur as a rare complication.

Remnants of the hyaloid artery are commonly associated with a persistent Bergmeister's papilla and/or with persistent hyperplastic primary vitreous; thus all three elements of the functional fetal vascular tree may persist and present as a congenital anomaly. Other ocular associations include optic disc coloboma, optic nerve hypoplasia and a posterior vitreous cyst.

Associated systemic features

None known.

Differential diagnosis

A hyaloid artery which contains blood has to be distinguished from:

1. A prepapillary vessel loop; and
2. Other abnormal vessels on the optic disc.

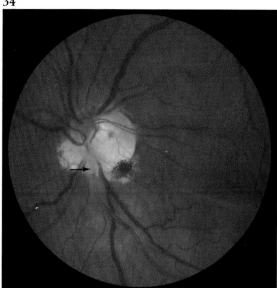

34 Persistent hyaloid artery seen as a semi-transparent remnant (arrow) overlying the inferior retinal vessels. There is an associated inferior coloboma of the optic disc with two areas of juxtapapillary pigmentary disturbance.

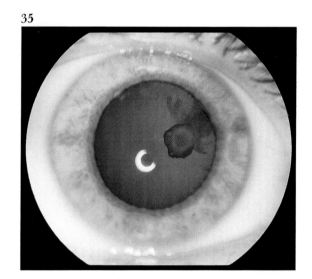

35 Mittendorf's dot showing as a dark opacity in the pupil against the red reflex of the fundus.

Persistent Bergmeister's papilla

Incomplete regression of the glial and fibrous tissue which forms the substance of Bergmeister's papilla leaves a remnant of variable size and density extending forwards from the optic disc; the physiological cup is consequently diminished or absent (*see* page 20).

Ophthalmoscopy (Fig. **36**)

1. Remnants of Bergmeister's papilla may present either as a faint grey veil overlying the structures of the optic disc, or may appear as a solid protruberance from the disc, yellow–white in colour and with a shiny, reflective surface.
2. Ninety per cent of such remnants are situated nasally on the disc.
3. The physiological optic cup is reduced or absent.

Supplementary findings

This non-progressive condition is generally asymptomatic and discovered in the course of a routine eye examination. Visual acuity is usually good, unless there are other associated

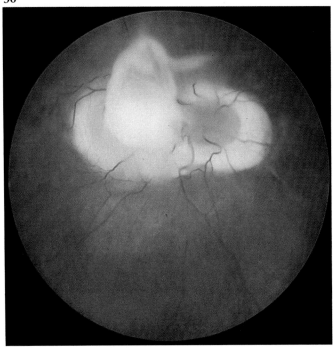

36 Persistent Bergmeister's papilla protruding from a colobomatous optic disc.

developmental abnormalities leading to visual deficit.

A coloboma may occur, as well as the expected ocular associations of persistent hyaloid artery and persistent hyperplastic primary vitreous, or prepapillary vascular loops.

Associated systemic features

None known.

Prepapillary vascular loops

Prepapillary vascular loops are thought to arise during the fetal period from aberrant mesodermal tissue within Bergmeister's papilla (*see* page 20). This tissue differentiates to form an anomalous vessel loop extending from the optic disc and linking two branches of the definitive central retinal vessels. The glial and fibrous tissue of Bergmeister's papilla may persist postnatally and remain associated with the vascular loop, or it may regress normally, when the loop appears to float freely in the vitreous.

Differential diagnosis

Persistent Bergmeister's papilla needs to be distinguished from:

1. Persistent hyperplastic primary vitreous.
2. The morning glory optic disc, to which it bears a superficial resemblance.
3. Conditions presenting as a pale, swollen or distorted optic disc.

Ninety-five per cent of prepapillary vessel loops originate from branches of the retinal arteries and 5 per cent from the veins; arterial and venous loops are rarely seen in the same eye. The condition generally occurs unilaterally (85 per cent of cases).

Ophthalmoscopy
(Fig. **37**)

1. Arterial loops may be short and simple, or they may be long with several spiral twists, resembling a corkscrew. They never reach

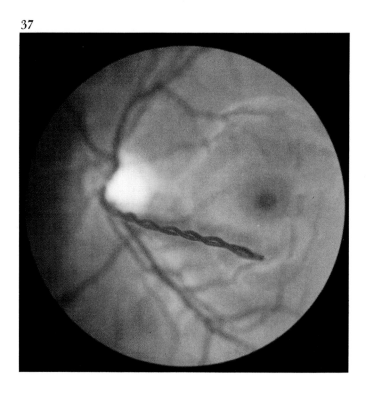

37 Prepapillary arterial loop, floating in the vitreous.

the posterior surface of the lens (cf. persistent hyaloid artery).

2. A loop usually originates from, and returns to, vessels on the optic disc, although occasionally an arterial loop may arise from an artery on the disc and return to a retinal branch.
3. Thirty per cent of arterial loops are surrounded by a white sheath, representing the residue of Bergmeister's papilla.
4. Unsupported loops may extend into the vitreous and change position with eye movements.
5. Arterial loops, which may pulsate, generally affect inferior central retinal vessels (70 per cent of cases), while venous loops usually affect superior retinal veins.

Supplementary findings

Prepapillary vessel loops are usually discovered on routine ophthalmological examination.

Arterial loops occasionally present with amaurosis fugax, or are complicated by retinal artery obstruction in that quadrant of the retina served by the arterial branch from which the loop derives. Vitreous haemorrhage and hyphaema have also been reported. Venous loops are not known to cause complications.

Cilioretinal arteries (*see* page 43) occur in about 75 per cent of cases with arterial loops.

Associated systemic features

None known.

Differential diagnosis

Prepapillary vascular loops should be differentiated from:

1. A persistent hyaloid artery.
2. Other abnormal vessels on the optic disc.

Persistent hyperplastic primary vitreous

Failure of regression of the embryonic or primary vitreous is followed by its hyperplasia, affecting both fibrous and vascular components. Even though the amount of primary vitreous tissue that remains postnatally is small in relation to the volume of the definitive vitreous, it is sufficient to cause abnormalities that are clinically significant. In more than half of cases, persistent hyperplastic primary vitreous (PHPV) is associated with remnants of the hyaloid arterial system.

The condition occurs unilaterally in 90 per cent of cases, the affected eye invariably being microphthalmic. PHPV presents as (i) a posterior form, related to the optic disc; and (ii) a more common anterior form, related to the lens: these are considered separately.

(i) Posterior form

Ophthalmoscopy

A pale, irregular membrane extends over the optic disc (Fig. **38**); it may distort the underlying retinal vessels, and stress lines, or traction lines, often develop in the retina. The membrane may be associated with remnants of Bergmeister's papilla, the hyaloid artery and/or a falciform retinal fold (Fig. **39**). The latter, comprising a fibrovascular band of primary vitreous, extends from the disc in any meridian to form a characteristic, crescentic fold.

Supplementary findings

Visual acuity is variable, but is usually poor from birth. There may be permanent loss of vision due to vitreous haemorrhage or retinal detachment.

The presence of a falciform retinal fold extending forwards from the optic disc to the ciliary region may predispose the lens to subluxation.

Associated systemic features

None known.

(ii) Anterior form

Ophthalmoscopy

1. Ophthalmoscopic examination may be difficult owing to the presence of a retrolental fibrous membrane or mass of tissue, representing the PHPV, which obscures the fundus view. A retrolental white pupillary reflex (leukocoria) is an important clinical sign, especially in an infant or child.
2. Traction on the ciliary body may cause the ciliary body processes to be drawn centripetally so that they can be seen within the pupil, around the circumference of the lens. This sign assists diagnosis.

Supplementary findings

Swelling of the cataractous lens may cause acute glaucoma, the latter aggravated by the commonly associated microphthalmia and shallow anterior chamber. Posterior synechiae may develop and present as iris bombé. In cases of long-standing glaucoma the microphthalmic eye may stretch, even becoming buphthalmic.

Associated systemic features

None known.

Differential diagnosis

1. The posterior form of PHPV should be distinguished from those abnormalities associated with a distorted, pale optic disc.
2. The differential diagnosis for anterior PHPV is that for leukocoria and comprises retinoblastoma, congenital cataract and retinopathy of prematurity (retrolental fibroplasia). The latter abnormality—a potential complication of oxygen administration to the premature infant—invariably develops bilaterally and causes dragging of the disc vessels (*see* page 42).

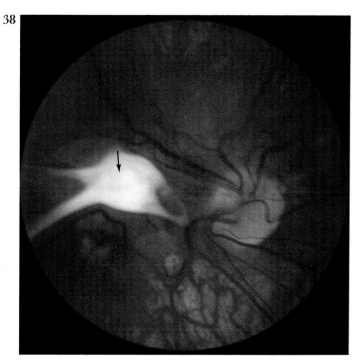

38 Persistent hyperplastic primary vitreous (posterior form). An irregular pale membrane near the optic disc (arrow) distorts the central retinal vessels as they emerge from the optic disc.

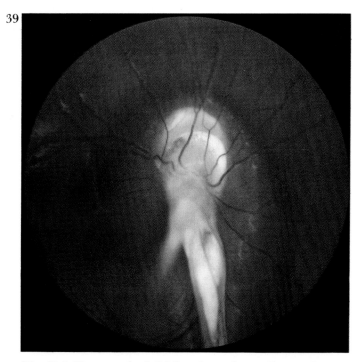

39 Falciform retinal fold and persistent Bergmeister's papilla associated with the posterior form of PHPV.

Other congenital vascular anomalies

Situs inversus

Situs inversus denotes an anomalous course of the retinal vessels as they emerge from the optic disc. In this congenital condition the temporal vessels first turn nasally, away from the macula, before curving temporally (cf. the normal, in which they pass directly to the temporal quadrants which they supply or drain). Embryologically, situs inversus is thought to be the outcome of dysversion—or tilting—of the optic disc and physiological optic cup, the central axis of the cup being directed nasally and thus changing the orientation of the temporal vessels.

Situs inversus occurs bilaterally in about 80 per cent of cases and is commonly a feature of the tilted disc syndrome. Thus the presence of situs inversus signals the possible coexistence of a tilted disc and should alert to the clinical significance of any temporal visual field defects (*see* page 24).

Ophthalmoscopy

1. The temporal vessels emerge nasally and then turn temporally, so that the nasal portion of the optic disc appears crowded and the physiological cup may be difficult to define (Fig. **40**).
2. Features of the commonly associated tilted disc syndrome may be observed (*see* page 24).
3. There may also be associated myopic changes, including a scleral crescent (*see* page 70).
4. Cilioretinal vessels are another common finding (*see* page 43).

Supplementary findings

Situs inversus, as the sole fundus abnormality, is not usually linked with any visual disturbance. However, temporal field defects and bitemporal hemianopia may occur in association with the tilted disc syndrome.

Associated systemic features

None known.

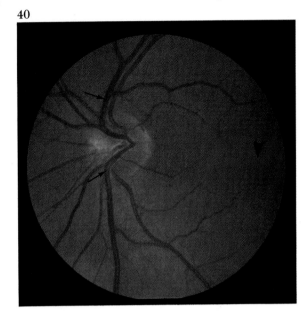

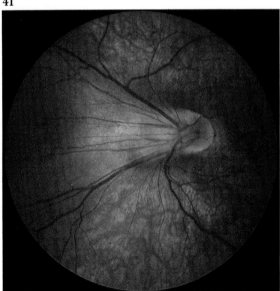

40 Situs inversus. The temporal vessels (arrows) emerge nasally from the optic disc before turning temporally towards the macula (triangle).

41 Dragged disc vessels mimic situs inversus. They are pathognomic of retinopathy of prematurity (retrolental fibroplasia, *see* page 40).

Differential diagnosis

Situs inversus has to be differentiated from other conditions in which the retinal vessels take an abnormal course (dragged vessels) (Fig. **41**).

Cilioretinal vessels

Although usually classified as a congenital anomaly, cilioretinal vessels should probably be considered a variant of the normal retinal vascular pattern. Cilioretinal arteries arise from the posterior ciliary circulation and extend forwards into the optic disc (*see* page 14). They are present in about 40 per cent of the population while cilioretinal veins occur only rarely.

Cilioretinal vessels emerge from, or enter the optic disc at its margin; they are associated with the choroidal circulation and are quite distinct from that of the central retinal arteries and veins. A cilioretinal artery (more than one is quite often present) usually lies on the temporal side of the optic disc and supplies the inner layers of the retina; 10 per cent supply the perifoveolar capillary network.

Ophthalmoscopy
(Figs. **42**, **43**)

1. Cilioretinal vessels usually lie on the temporal side of the optic disc (90 per cent of cases), emerging or entering from the disc margin or adjacent peripapillary area.
2. The are often hook-shaped at the margin of the disc.
3. Although many of them traverse the macular area, only a small proportion (10 per cent) of cilioretinal arteries supply the perifoveolar capillaries.

Supplementary findings

The clinical significance of a cilioretinal blood supply becomes apparent in the event of a central retinal artery occlusion (Figs. **44** and **45**) when—in the presence of a cilioretinal artery—the macular area may be spared and vision maintained. Conversely, in those individuals in whom a cilioretinal artery supplies the macula, occlusion of this vessel may result in loss of central vision.

The prevalence of cilioretinal arteries is increased in patients with congenital optic disc pits, prepapillary arterial loops, optic disc drusen and situs inversus.

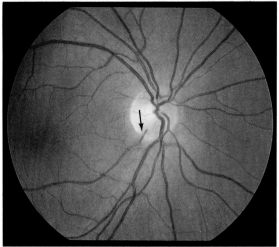

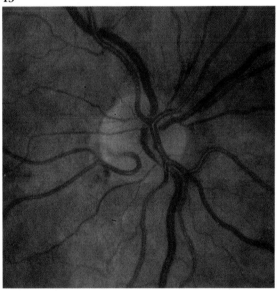

42 Cilioretinal artery (arrow) emerging from the temporal area of the optic disc.

43 Cilioretinal artery showing the typical hook-shaped origin.

Systemic associations
None known.

Differential diagnosis

Cilioretinal vessels have to be differentiated from other abnormal vessels on the optic disc.

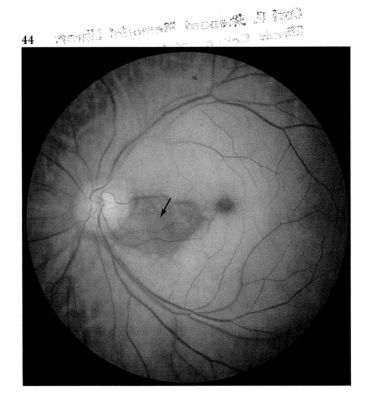

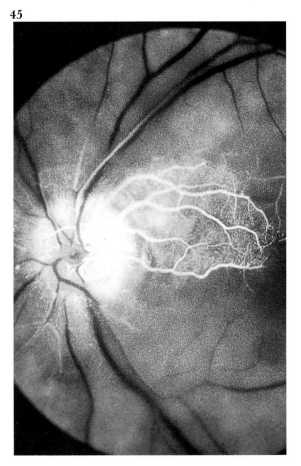

44 A central retinal artery occlusion has resulted in a pale, oedematous retina, with the exception of the papillomacular area (arrow) where the retinal circulation is maintained by cilioretinal vessels. A 'cherry-red spot' at the macula (in the foveolar region, free of retinal ganglion cells) signifies an intact underlying choroidal circulation.

45 Fundus fluorescein angiogram of the case illustrated in Fig. **44**, showing delayed perfusion of the central retinal vessels; this contrasts with the well-perfused cilioretinal circulation extending from the temporal margin of the optic disc.

Tortuosity of retinal vessels

Congenital tortuosity involves retinal arteries more commonly than retinal veins. The normally sinuous course of vessels leaving the optic disc is exaggerated; the condition occurs bilaterally and affects all four quadrants of the fundus. Congenital tortuosity of the retinal vessels is non-progressive, except in instances of the rare entity known as progressive congenital arteriolar tortuosity, inherited in an autosomal dominant pattern.

Ophthalmoscopy

1. In non-progressive congenital tortuosity both arteries and veins may be affected, but their colour and calibre are normal and there are no other vascular changes (Fig. **46**).
2. In the progressive, autosomal-dominant type, the medium-sized and smaller retinal arterioles are affected exclusively, most noticeably in the macular area; associated retinal haemorrhages may be visible.

Supplementary findings

Non-progressive congenital tortuosity of the retinal vessels is symptomless and usually discovered on routine eye examination. Hypermetropia may be an associated finding.

Progressive congenital retinal tortuosity may present with visual symptoms caused by spontaneous retinal haemorrhages. As the vascular tortuosity may not become obvious until early adolescence, when it progresses markedly, the diagnosis may be missed during childhood. Examination of older members of the family may help to establish the diagnosis and thus prevent unnecessary haematological and cardiological investigation of these patients.

Associated systemic features

None known.

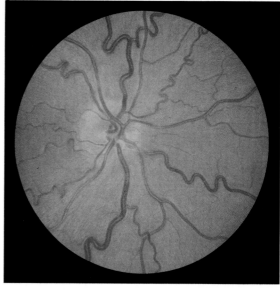

46   Congenital tortuosity of the retinal veins.

Differential diagnosis

Congenital tortuosity of the retinal vessels should be differentiated from:

1. Collateral vessels.
2. Tortuosity arising secondary to local ocular or generalized systemic disorders; these include retinal vein occlusion, diabetic retinopathy, coarctation of the aorta and congenital heart disease.

Retinal macrovessels

In this congenital vascular anomaly, an enlarged but otherwise normal blood vessel can be seen entering or leaving the optic disc and traversing the retina. Veins are affected more often than arteries (in the ratio 3:1) and the anomaly usually occurs unilaterally. A retinal macrovessel is thought to arise during the differentiation of major vessels from the primitive capillary network, when one 'channel' or vessel enlarges preferentially, probably in response to haemodynamic factors.

Ophthalmoscopy

1. A single enlarged vessel extends transversely from the optic disc and crosses the macular region; it has branches subserving both the superior and inferior quadrants of the temporal retina (Fig. **47**).

2. Adjacent retinal vessels tend to be small and displaced away from the macrovessel and its tributaries.

3. The fovea may be ectopically placed and/or contain a foveal cyst.

Supplementary findings

Visual acuity is usually normal; a macrovessel is generally an incidental finding at routine ophthalmological examination. Even when a foveal cyst is present, visual acuity is only minimally reduced.

Associated systemic features

None known.

Differential diagnosis

A retinal macrovessel has to be differentiated from other conditions involving enlargement of blood vessels in the papillary region; in particular, it should be distinguished from racemose haemangioma.

47

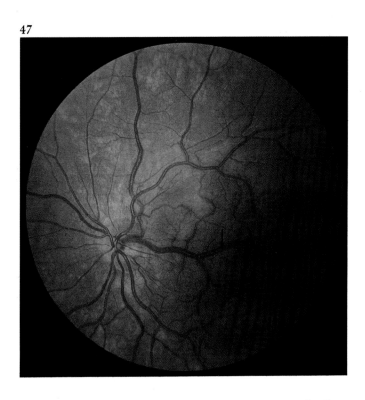

47 A retinal macrovessel courses from the optic disc across the macula (arrow).

Racemose haemangioma
(Circoid haemangioma)

Racemose haemangiomas, like retinal macro-vessels, are thought to arise as a result of aberrant vascular remodelling during the process of formation of definitive retinal vessels from the early capillary network. These haemangiomas represent an arteriovenous shunt, with absence of intervening capillary elements. Thus pressure within the arteries and veins is equalized, with the result that both vessel types are dilated and appear similar in calibre and colour as they traverse the retina, leaving and returning to the optic disc. This rare condition almost always occurs unilaterally.

Classically, racemose haemangiomas are divided into three grades of increasing severity. The first grade is mild and vessel enlargement is localized whereas, in the third grade, the whole of the optic disc and much of the fundus may be obscured by a network of dilated, tortuous vessels; the second grade is an intermediate state. The second and third grades of retinal involvement are associated with intracranial and facial vascular disorders; they show a dominant inheritance pattern, forming part of the Wyburn–Mason syndrome.

Ophthalmoscopy

1. The degree of involvement of retinal vessels varies from mild to severe, with one or more large, dilated vessels running a tortuous course across the retina; afferent and efferent limbs of the vessel loop exit and enter from the optic disc, but arterial and venous sections are difficult to distinguish, being the same colour and calibre (the latter may be uneven) (Fig. **48**).
2. One of more quadrants of the optic disc, or the whole optic disc, may be obscured, together with part or much of the fundus.
3. Retinal exudates occur only rarely.

48

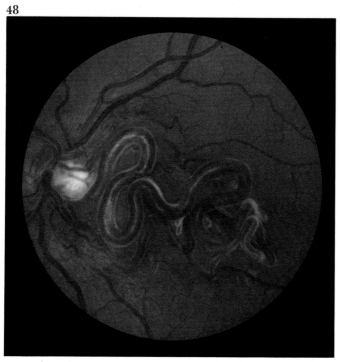

48   A racemose haemangioma.

Supplementary findings

This is a non-progressive retinal disorder. The mild form may be asymptomatic and an incidental finding on routine eye examination. However, physical exertion may precipitate retinal haemorrhages (Fig. **49**) and produce transient scotomas. The extreme grade is associated with severe visual loss if the vessels, which extend over a large part of the fundus, also overlie the macula. Additional ocular complications, associated with the Wyburn–Mason syndrome, may be present (*see* below).

Fluorescein angiography classically shows a rapid transit time due to the absence of a capillary bed between retinal arterioles and venules. Leakage of dye occurs rarely and then only from those vessels that are grossly enlarged.

Associated systemic features

Computerized tomography may be indicated in order to investigate for associated features of the Wyburn–Mason syndrome. These occur in 75 per cent of cases in which retinal involvement is severe; they include ipsilateral vascular anomalies of the brain, face and orbit. Maxillo-mandibular anomalies carry the risk of severe haemorrhage as a complication of dental extraction. Eye movements may be affected by brain stem lesions involving the nuclei of the 3rd, 4th or 6th cranial nerves. There may be epilepsy or spontaneous cerebral haemorrhage.

Differential diagnosis

Racemose haemangioma should be distinguished from:

1. Other enlarged vessels originating from the optic disc.
2. Other conditions in which vascular masses overlie the optic disc.

49

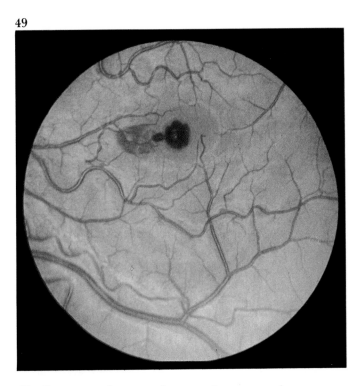

49 Racemose haemangioma, a less severe form, complicated by retinal haemorrhage.

Acquired vascular abnormalities

Retinal artery occlusion

An occlusion may occur in any part of the retinal arterial system. Occlusions occurring at or near the optic disc affect vision more severely than those in the peripheral retina.

One of three mechanisms may be responsible for an occlusion in the retinal arterial system. Of these, emboli from the heart or atheromatous large vessels are probably the most common; septic emboli may arise as a result of intravenous drug abuse. Emboli are particularly likely to become lodged either at the lamina cribrosa, causing central retinal artery occlusion, or at the bifurcation of an arteriolar branch in the retina. Less frequently the vessel lumen may be narrowed or obliterated, and blood flow restricted, by intrinsic changes in the vessel wall. These include atheroma or inflammatory disorders, such as giant cell arteritis. Arterial occlusion may also result from a sudden rise in intraocular pressure caused by acute angle-closure glaucoma, or produced by inadvertent pressure on the eye during ophthalmic or neurosurgical procedures.

Ophthalmoscopy

The changes that occur after retinal arterial occlusion may be divided into those of the acute phase, and the long-term sequelae.

In the acute phase (Figs. **50, 51**):

1. Initially the occluded vessel may be narrowed and darkened (owing to stasis and sludging of the blood); the blood column may be segmented, giving a 'rail-truck' appearance. These changes are transitory and may last for only a few hours.
2. The retina which is in the area of distribution of the occluded artery is grey-white and opaque, due to retinal oedema.
3. In instances where the central retinal artery is occluded, the foveola, which derives its blood supply from the underlying choroid, retains its normal colour, giving rise to the classic 'cherry-red spot'. This sign becomes apparent after a few hours and persists for about 2 weeks. If a cilioretinal artery is

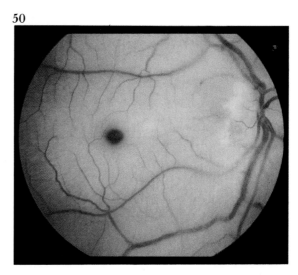

50

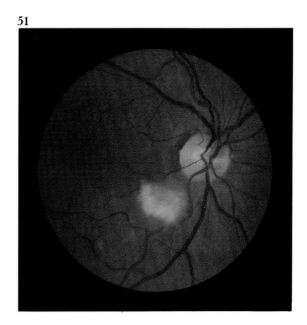

51

50   Central retinal artery occlusion. The retina is pale and oedematous and there is a 'cherry-red spot' at the macula.

51   Branch retinal artery occlusion, resulting in a localized, pale area of retinal infarction.

present, the papillomacular bundle may be spared (*see* page 43).
4. An embolus may be visible within an occluded vessel, most often lodged at a bifurcation (Fig. **52**).

49

In the long term (Fig. **53**):

1. A previously occluded artery may have re-opened by the time a patient is examined, in which case it will appear thread-like and may show fibrotic sheathing.
2. The normal fundus colour returns as the retinal oedema subsides.
3. Arterial collateral vessels occasionally develop (*see* page 56).

Supplementary findings

The hallmark of retinal arterial occlusion is a sudden, painless loss of vision which may be either permanent or, if small emboli are involved, merely transient (amaurosis fugax). The extent of the visual loss is dependent upon both the size and location of the vessel affected: thus occlusion of a small vessel at the macula will severely affect visual acuity, whereas occlusion of a vessel of similar size, but situated in the peripheral retina, may be asymptomatic. Visual field loss is characteristically segmental. An afferent pupillary defect may be present in more severe cases.

Retinal neovascularization and rubeosis of the iris are rare complications (less than 2 per cent of cases) but may arise within a few weeks (cf. retinal vein occlusion, *see* page 52).

Associated systemic features

There may be a clinical history and physical evidence of vascular insufficiency caused by one of several aetiological factors: for example, atherosclerosis or hypertension. The presence of arterial occlusion is an indication for urgent referral since it may reflect serious cardio-vascular pathology. In addition, other systemic disorders such as hyperlipidaemia, haemo-globinopathies and various causes of vasculitis (autoimmune disease, secondary syphilis) need to be considered.

Differential diagnosis

Retinal arterial occlusion has to be differentiated from other types of vascular occlusion involving the optic disc.

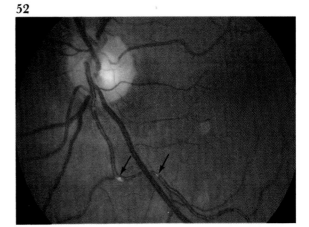

52

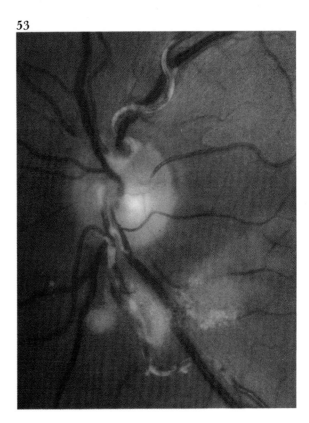

53

52   Two emboli at the bifurcations of a retinal arteriole (arrows); small emboli may be only transient.

53   Long-standing central retinal artery occlusion. The retinal arteries have partially re-opened but show fibrotic sheathing.

Retinal vein occlusion

Venous occlusion is one of the most common retinal vascular disorders. Occlusion of the central retinal vein occurs chiefly at the lamina cribrosa, whereas branch vein occlusion most commonly takes place at an arteriovenous crossing where arteriole and venule share a common connective-tissue sheath. The venule is therefore particularly susceptible to pressure exerted at the crossing by a thickened arteriole, as may occur in arteriosclerosis or hypertension (*see* page 14). Several other factors, involving either local ocular disorders or systemic disease, can play an aetiological role in retinal venous occlusion. The former category includes raised intraocular pressure caused by primary chronic glaucoma, or by secondary glaucoma associated with intraocular inflammation. In addition, space-occupying lesions in the orbit may cause retrobulbar compression and inhibit venous return. Systemic disorders associated with retinal vein occlusion include hypertension, hyperlipidaemia, hyperviscosity of the blood (e.g. polycythaemia, chronic leukaemia), vasculitis (e.g. sarcoidosis, Behçet's disease) and, possibly, diabetes mellitus.

There are three types of retinal venous occlusion, which are age related; all show similar changes in the fundus, but vary in severity. In the younger age group (15–30 years), central retinal vein occlusion gives rise to the condition known as *papillophlebitis* (Fig. **54**). Patients are healthy, with no associated systemic disease, such as hypertension. The prognosis for visual acuity is usually good. The two other variants of central retinal vein occlusion occur in older patients; they are *venous stasis retinopathy* (Fig. **55**) and *haemorrhagic venous occlusion* (Fig. **56**). Venous stasis retinopathy accompanies arteriosclerotic changes and is characterized by venous dilatation and tortuosity, flame-shaped retinal haemorrhages and a few cotton-wool infarcts. Chronic macular oedema is a common complication, leading to a permanent reduction in central visual acuity. Haemorrhagic venous occlusion, on the other hand, is characterized by extensive retinal haemorrhages and numerous cotton-wool infarcts, denoting severe retinal ischaemia (Fig. **57**). The prognosis is poor because of serious ocular complications (*see* below).

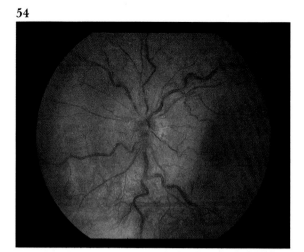

54

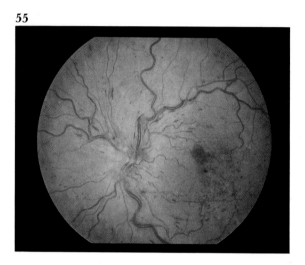

55

54 Papillophlebitis. The optic disc is swollen and the retinal veins distended.

55 Central retinal vein occlusion (venous stasis type). The retinal veins are distended; there are a few flame-shaped retinal haemorrhages scattered through the fundus, with a large haemorrhage at the macula.

Ophthalmoscopy

As in instances of retinal artery occlusion, the changes that occur after retinal vein occlusion may be divided into those of the acute phase, and the long-term sequelae.

In the acute phase:

1. Extravasated blood collects in the retina, forming deep and superficial haemorrhages. In cases of branch vein occlusion the

haemorrhages are localized, but when the central retinal vein is blocked, multiple haemorrhages give rise to the dramatic fundus picture known as 'sunset' or 'battlefield' fundus.

2. Peripheral to the site of occlusion the venous channels are dilated and tortuous and the blood column is darkened, owing to stasis.

3. The optic disc is swollen and congested and has ill-defined margins, caused by oedema of both the disc and retina; these changes may affect a segment of the disc (branch vein occlusion, Fig. **58**), or the whole disc (central retinal vein occlusion). In the latter case, spontaneous venous pulsation (normally best seen at the disc) is absent.

4. Cotton-wool spots (nerve fibre layer infarcts) reflect severe retinal ischaemia and are associated with haemorrhagic retinal vein occlusion.

In the long-standing phase:

1. Blood may have been resorbed from the retina and venous collateral vessels may have developed, by-passing the obstruction. Collateral vessels occur either locally in the retina or, in the case of central retinal vein occlusion, in the optic nerve head (*see* Fig. **69**). Their distended, tortuous appearance helps to distinguish them from new vessels, which usually form a lace-like network (*see* page 54).

2. The walls of occluded vessels may appear pale due to fibrotic sheathing.

3. Chronic oedema may result in pigmentary change at the macula.

Supplementary findings

Visual loss is painless and occurs slowly (cf. retinal arterial occlusion). In papillophlebitis the patient may notice visual blurring which progresses over several hours or days. The haemorrhagic form of the disorder may develop so slowly that the patient becomes aware of visual loss only when inadvertently occluding the fellow eye.

In instances of central retinal vein occlusion the visual field shows a central scotoma with peripheral field constriction; with branch vein occlusion the field loss is segmental. There may be an afferent pupillary defect, related to the extent of retinal damage. In cases associated with chronic glaucoma there may be a transient lowering of intraocular pressure in the eye affected by the occlusion, in contrast to the raised intraocular pressure in the fellow eye. It is therefore essential, at examination, to check the pressure in both eyes.

Haemorrhagic central retinal vein occlusion may be complicated by neovascularization of the retina and optic disc, as well as of the iris (rubeosis; Figs. **59**, **60**). New vessels on the retina and optic disc frequently result in further visual impairment due to vitreous haemorrhage. Rubeosis of the iris invariably leads to neovascular glaucoma, described as 'hundred-day glaucoma' since it usually arises within about 3 months of the venous occlusion. Although some retinal neovascularization may be associated with branch vein occlusion, rubeosis of the iris rarely occurs. These complications can often be avoided by retinal laser photocoagulation, provided it is applied sufficiently early.

Differential diagnosis

Three categories need to be considered:

1. Other types of vascular occlusion involving the optic disc.

2. Conditions presenting with retinal haemorrhage and tortuosity of the retinal blood vessels (e.g. diabetes mellitus, congenital tortuosity of the retinal vessels).

3. Conditions in which the optic disc is hyperaemic and swollen.

56

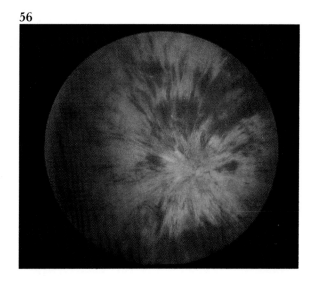

57

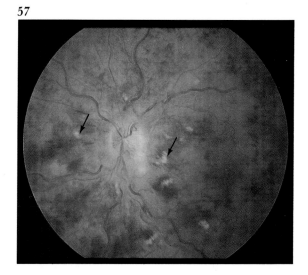

58

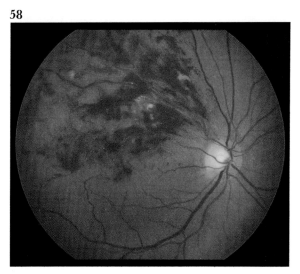

59

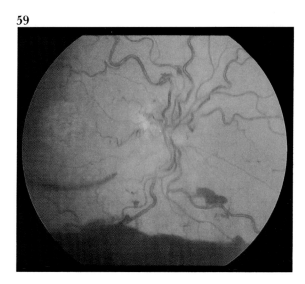

60

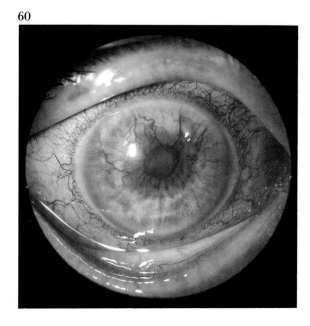

56 Haemorrhagic central retinal vein occlusion. Multiple retinal haemorrhages almost entirely obscure the tortuous, engorged retinal vessels.

57 Cotton-wool spots (arrows), a sign of retinal ischaemia, are often associated with haemorrhagic retinal vein occlusion.

58 Retinal branch vein occlusion.

59 New vessels on the optic disc, a complication of central retinal vein occlusion. The fundus view is hazy owing to vitreous haemorrhage, with pooling of blood inferiorly.

60 Rubeosis of the iris. New vessels extend radially over the anterior surface of the iris and pass into the pupil.

New vessels on the optic disc

The formation of new vessels on the optic disc is the hallmark of diabetic retinopathy in its proliferative stage. The new vessels are usually asymptomatic but, if the condition is allowed to progress, vitreous haemorrhage and loss of vision ensue. Diabetic retinopathy is one of the most common causes of blindness amongst the working-age population in industrialized countries. Recognition of new vessels on the optic disc during fundus examination is therefore of vital importance, since urgent referral of the patient for laser photocoagulation is essential at this stage, if the treatment is to be effective and blindness prevented.

In addition to diabetic retinopathy, other conditions characterized by retinal ischaemia may also show neovascularization (*see under* retinal artery occlusion, page 49; retinal vein occlusion, page 51).

Ophthalmoscopy
(Figs. **61–64**)

1. A fine network of vessels can be seen on the optic disc; the network may either lie flat on the disc or protrude into the vitreous; it may cover just a segment of the disc, or the whole of it, even extending onto the adjacent retina. New vessels in the network further differ from the main retinal vessels on the optic disc in that they do not branch dichotomously.
2. There may be associated neovascularization in the adjacent and/or peripheral retina.
3. The new vessels are likely to break and bleed, leading to preretinal or vitreous haemorrhage.
4. Other features related to the aetiology should be sought for in the fundus of the same eye

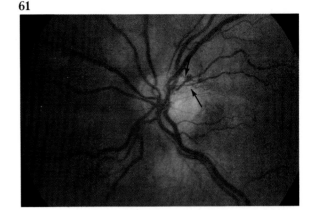

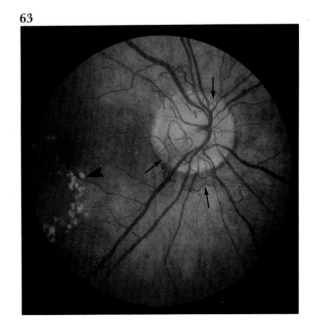

61 **A small cluster of new vessels on the optic disc** (arrows).

62 **New vessels;** these extend from the optic disc into the adjacent retina in two fan-like networks (arrows).

63 **Diabetic retinopathy.** There are new vessels on the optic disc and retina (arrows) and hard exudates (triangle) at the macula.

and in the contralateral eye. In diabetic retinopathy, for example, these include microaneurysms, dot and blot retinal haemorrhages, hard exudates and cotton-wool infarcts.

Supplementary findings

New vessels are asymptomatic, until they break and bleed, when the patient may complain of seeing 'floaters', commonly described as being like 'tadpoles' or 'spiders' webs'; severe visual loss may occur suddenly owing to haemorrhage into the vitreous. This may eventually clear spontaneously, but long-term vitreous haemorrhage can result in organization of the vitreous, with dragging of the retinal vessels and traction retinal detachment (Figs. **65**, **66**).

As well as new vessels, other signs and symptoms of the underlying aetiology may present in the fundus. In addition, cases of severe retinal ischaemia (from whatever cause) may be complicated by rubeosis of the iris and neovascular glaucoma.

Fundus fluorescein angiography shows a characteristic pattern (Fig. **67**), which helps to distinguish new vessels from collateral vessels (*see* page 56). New vessels fill early in the arterial phase and leak dye profusely; collateral vessels only rarely leak dye.

Associated systemic features

Systemic features are those related to the aetiology of the primary disorder.

Differential diagnosis

New vessels have to be distinguished from other conditions in which:

1. There are abnormal vessels, or
2. Vessel masses on the optic disc.
3. Vessels on the optic disc appear dragged.

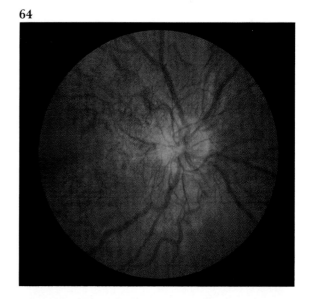

64 Extensive neovascularization with a moderate degree of associated fibrosis.

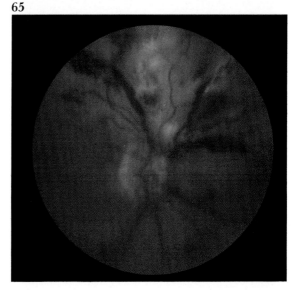

65 A vitreous haemorrhage obscuring most of the fundus detail in a case of diabetic retinopathy.

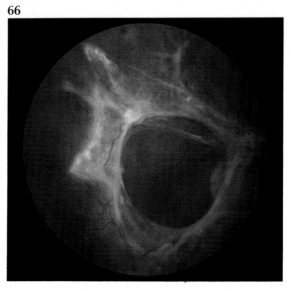

66 Advanced diabetic retinopathy. Fibrotic organization of a vitreous haemorrhage has resulted in dragging of the disc vessels and traction retinal detachment.

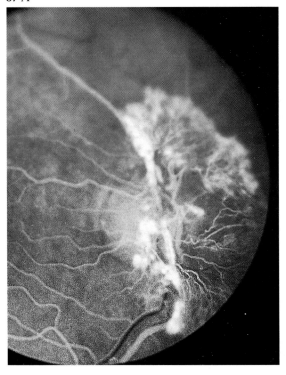

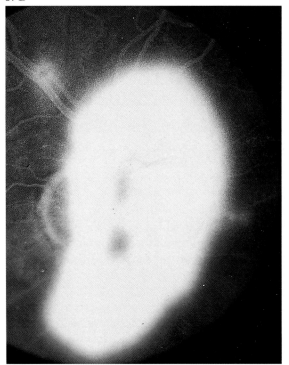

67 Fundus fluorescein angiogram of new vessels (the patient had secondary syphilis). (**A**) Early stage: the network of new vessels on the optic disc is filled with dye. (**B**) Late stage: profuse leakage of dye obscures the optic disc.

Collateral vessels

Collateral vessels arise, not as a primary abnormality of the retinal vascular system, but in response to stasis or occlusion which may take place on either the venous or arterial side of the intraocular circulation. Their presence is therefore indicative of a preceding retinovascular disorder which may, in turn, signify an underlying ocular or systemic disease requiring investigation.

Collateral vessels originate from already established minor vessels which expand to compensate for functional insufficiency in an adjacent major vessel; they form a new link between pre-existing arterial or venous channels. Although distorted and dilated, collateral vessels branch dichotomously and retain the normal architectural pattern of the vascular tree (cf. the intricate network of vessels characteristic of neovascularization, *see* page 54).

Depending on the site of occlusion of the main vessel, collateral vessels may occur locally in the retina, in the juxtapapillary region, or on the optic disc.

Ophthalmoscopy

1. Collateral vessels are dilated and tortuous and form a link between two elements of the retinal arterial or venous circulations, bypassing the defective sector of the occluded vessel (Fig. **68**).
2. Alternatively, collateral vessels may link retinal vessels with the choroidal circulation. In this instance they form a short, hook-like loop at the point where they penetrate the retina or optic disc, giving rise to retinociliary or opticociliary shunt vessels (*see* Fig. **122**), respectively.
3. The 'ghost' remnant of the occluded vessel is often discernible.

Differential diagnosis

Correct identification of collateral vessels is important, for the following reasons:

1. They must be distinguished from new vessels because patients with the latter condition require early referral for treatment by laser photocoagulation (*see* page 54); collateral vessels should never be photocoagulated as this will render them non-functional.

2. Since collateral vessels often constitute the only evidence of a previous vascular occlusion (Fig. **69**), their recognition should stimulate investigations into the aetiology of the primary systemic disorder (*see* retinal artery occlusion, page 49; retinal vein occlusion, page 51).

3. Similarly, collateral vessels are often the only evidence of a compromised intraocular blood supply, caused by a disease process outside the globe (e.g. a meningioma, *see* page 97).

4. Collateral vessels also have to be distinguished from other abnormal vascular structures in the eye. These may be non-progressive and innocent (e.g. congenital retinal macrovessels, *see* page 46). Alternatively, they may be associated with tumours requiring urgent investigation and treatment (e.g. capillary haemangioma, *see* page 92; retinoblastoma, *see* page 98).

68

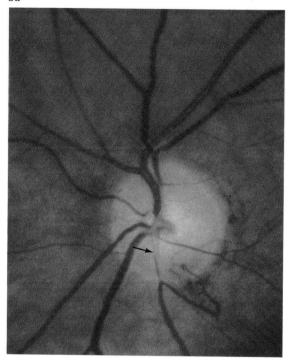

68   A U-shaped collateral vessel bypassing an obstructed branch of the central retinal artery, seen as an attenuated 'ghost' vessel (arrow).

69   Central retinal vein occlusion resulting in collateral vessel formation. (**A**) Central retinal vein occlusion, acute stage. (**B**) The same case, a few months later. The retinal haemorrhages have been absorbed; however, the distended collateral vessels on the optic disc provide a useful clue to the preceding pathology.

69 A

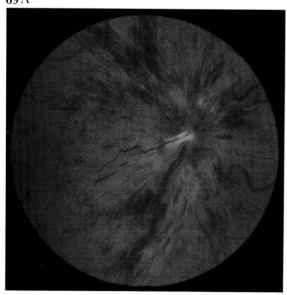

69 B

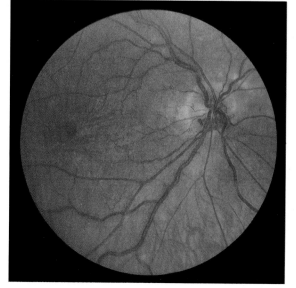

4: Optic Neuritis and Optic Neuropathy

The terms optic neuritis and optic neuropathy refer to abnormalities affecting the optic nerve and/or the blood vessels that supply it. It is conventional to reserve the term optic neuritis for demyelinating or inflammatory conditions, and optic neuropathy for disorders involving ischaemia or toxicity.

The criteria used in the classification of optic neuritis and optic neuropathy are somewhat complex, being based upon: (i) the region of the optic nerve which is affected by pathological change, and (ii) the stage of progression of the disorder (i.e. acute *vs.* chronic stage) (Fig. **70**).

If the optic nerve is affected behind the globe, the condition is called *retrobulbar neuritis* (or *retrobulbar neuropathy*). In the early phase the disc is normal in appearance; in the late stage there is *primary optic atrophy*.

If the optic disc or nerve head is affected, the condition is known as *papillitis* (or *papillopathy*). In the early stage the disc is oedematous and the physiological cup filled in. At a later stage there is *secondary optic atrophy*.

If the ganglion cell layer of the retina is mainly involved, the condition is known as *neuroretinitis*. In the early phase there may be swelling of the optic disc and retinal nerve fibre layer; other changes may also occur in the fundus. Progression is to *consecutive optic atrophy*.

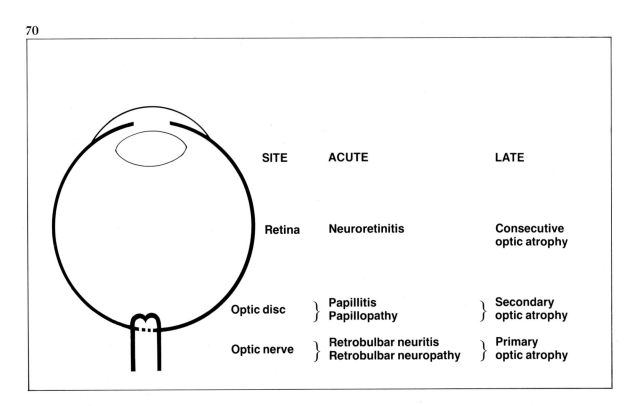

70   Terminology used to describe optic neuritis and optic neuropathy.

Optic neuritis

Optic neuritis may affect the optic nerve fibres in their retrobulbar portion, at the optic nerve head, or in the retinal ganglion cell layer. The aetiological factors are demyelination and inflammation.

Demyelination is most commonly caused by multiple sclerosis, or the variant of that condition named Devic's disease (neuromyelitis optica). Multiple sclerosis typically develops unilaterally, presenting between the ages of 20 and 45 years; it rarely appears after 60 years of age. Devic's disease characteristically occurs bilaterally in association with a transverse myelitis; it can affect any age group.

Inflammation may result from viral infection, granulomatous infective disorders such as syphilis, or the spread of infection from nearby meninges or sinuses.

Although all of these aetiological conditions may affect any part of the optic nerve, particular disorders show a regional predilection. Thus, for example, multiple sclerosis causes retrobulbar neuritis more often than it initiates papillitis or neuroretinitis.

Ophthalmoscopy

The appearance of the optic disc in optic neuritis varies, as follows:

1. In *retrobulbar neuritis* (Fig. **71**), in the early phase, the disc appears normal; later there is *primary optic atrophy* (*see* page 67).
2. In *papillitis* (Fig. **72**), in the early stage, the disc is moderately swollen and hyperaemic. There may be splinter haemorrhages on the surface of the disc and its margin may be indistinct. Progression is to *secondary optic atrophy* (*see* page 68).
3. In *neuroretinitis*, in the early stage, the optic disc may appear swollen but abnormal features in the surrounding retina are likely to be more in evidence. The latter may include an exudative macular star surrounding the fovea (more pronounced on the side towards the optic disc) and the appearance of inflammatory cells in the posterior vitreous. In the late phase there are signs of *consecutive optic atrophy* (*see* page 68).

Supplementary findings

Visual acuity usually decreases suddenly (i.e. within a period of 24 hours), its subsequent course being linked with the stage and nature of the causative disease. If, for example, optic neuritis is brought about by multiple sclerosis, the visual acuity may recover almost as rapidly. When associated with infective conditions, however, the decline in visual acuity is likely to be severe and permanent; it may be reduced to hand-movements only.

All cases of optic neuritis show an afferent pupillary defect, the extent of which correlates with the degree of visual loss. Various types of visual field defects are found, depending on the region of the optic nerve affected. Papillitis classically causes a central scotoma—a factor that assists its differentiation from optic disc swelling caused by papilloedema (*see* page 75). Optic neuritis also causes disturbances of colour vision; loss of red/green discrimination is typical of multiple sclerosis. In instances where there is retrobulbar neuritis, the patient may complain of mild discomfort on ocular movement.

Ocular symptoms and signs of multiple sclerosis are significant in that they may precede, by up to several years, other manifestations of the disease. There are two further ophthalmological symptoms which are characteristic of this disorder. The first is Uhthoff's phenomenon, in which visual acuity decreases as body temperature rises, so that patients typically complain that their visual acuity is reduced when, for example, they take a warm bath, or exercise. The second, Pulfrich's phenomenon, represents a disturbance in depth perception, particularly for moving objects. Thus, for example, a patient approaching an escalator may be unable to discern whether it is moving upwards or downwards.

Associated systemic features

These are related to the primary condition.

Differential diagnosis

1. The primary optic atrophy that follows retrobulbar neuritis has to be distinguished from other conditions in which the optic disc is pale and flat.
2. Papillitis has to be distinguished from other conditions in which the optic disc is hyperaemic and swollen.
3. Secondary optic atrophy (resulting from papillitis) has to be distinguished from other conditions in which the optic disc is pale and swollen.

71 A

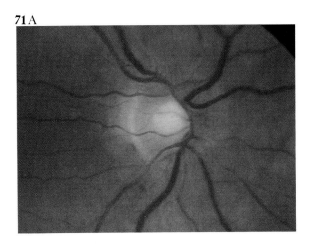

71 B

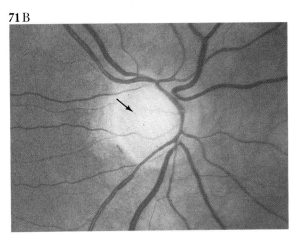

71 Retrobulbar neuritis. (**A**) The optic disc appears normal in the acute stage. (**B**) Later primary optic atrophy occurs which, in this case, is more marked on the temporal aspect of the disc (arrow).

72

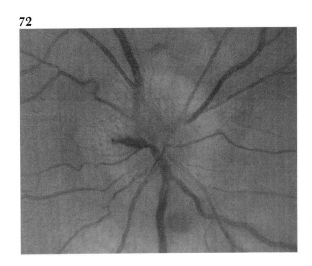

72 Papillitis. The disc is hyperaemic and moderately swollen and the disc margin is indistinct.

Optic neuropathy

In optic neuropathy, various disorders affect the optic nerve fibres along their course from the retina to the brain. As in optic neuritis, certain disease processes have a tendency to occur in the retrobulbar portion of the optic nerve, in the optic nerve head, or in the ganglion cells of the retina (*see* Fig. **70**). Aetiological factors include ischaemic and toxic conditions.

In ischaemic optic neuropathy the blood supply to the optic nerve and/or nerve head is compromised. Examples described in this section include idiopathic ischaemic optic neuropathy, giant cell arteritis (arteritic papillopathy) and diabetic papillopathy. For the sake of convenience, Leber's hereditary optic neuropathy is also considered; this condition is difficult to classify, but affects the peripapillary capillaries.

In the toxic optic neuropathies, the metabolism of the neural elements is affected by chemical agents, such as nicotine (in tobacco amblyopia) and other drugs (e.g. ethambutol and chloramphenicol), or by poisons (e.g. lead).

Idiopathic ischaemic optic neuropathy

Idiopathic ischaemic optic neuropathy is a common cause of sudden visual loss in elderly patients, with a peak incidence in the 60 to 70-year-old age group. It occurs as a result of ischaemic infarction in the optic nerve and nerve head. The short posterior ciliary arteries that supply the optic nerve, at and anterior to the lamina cribrosa, are particularly vulnerable to occlusion, giving rise to clinical features in which ischaemic papillopathy dominates.

Although atherosclerosis and carotid artery insufficiency are thought to be the main aetiological factors, hypertension may also be implicated.

Ophthalmoscopy

The presenting features differ according to the region of the optic nerve affected and the stage reached at the time of examination.

1. In *retrobulbar optic neuropathy*, in the early phase, the disc appears normal; later there is *primary optic atrophy* (*see* page 67).

73 Idiopathic ischaemic papillopathy. (**A**) In the acute phase the optic disc is pale and swollen, with splinter haemorrhages on the disc margin. (**B**) Later, secondary optic atrophy develops.

73 A

73 B

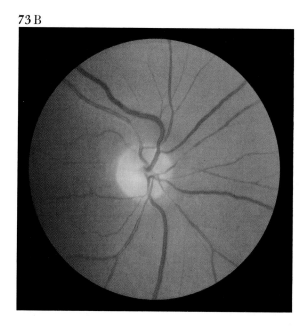

2. In *ischaemic papillopathy* (Fig. **73**), in the acute phase, the optic disc is swollen but pale; superficial splinter haemorrhages may be present on or near the disc. Cotton-wool infarcts commonly occur in the juxta-papillary region, and the juxtapapillary choroid may be pale. The central retinal vessels are often attenuated. In the chronic phase, *secondary optic atrophy* develops (*see* page 68).

Supplementary findings

Visual loss is rapid and painless, occurring unilaterally in the first instance. The second eye becomes involved in about 50 per cent of cases, after a lapse of months, or even years. This time-lag may give rise to the pseudo-Foster–Kennedy syndrome, in which there is optic atrophy in one eye and disc oedema in the other (*see also* papilloedema, page 75).

The visual deficit is usually moderate, but permanent, and always associated with an afferent pupillary defect. An altitudinal visual field defect is a classic finding.

Associated systemic features

These are related to atherosclerosis of the vascular system.

Differential diagnosis

1. The primary optic atrophy which follows retrobulbar optic neuropathy has to be differentiated from other conditions in which the optic disc is pale and flat.
2. Papillopathy, and the secondary optic atrophy that succeeds it, have to be differentiated from other conditions in which the optic disc is pale and swollen.

Giant cell arteritis
(Arteritic papillopathy)

Giant cell arteritis is an autoimmune disorder affecting patients over the age of 60 years. Inflammation of elastic tissue in the media and adventitia of arterial walls leads to vascular occlusion.

Inflammation in the superficial temporal arteries, and in arteries of similar calibre elsewhere in the body, results in a spectrum of characteristic clinical features. Concurrent involvement of the ophthalmic and posterior ciliary arteries causes ischaemic papillopathy, often presenting as unilateral loss of vision. Together these findings constitute a syndrome of major clinical significance; its prompt diagnosis and treatment with systemic steroids can prevent blindness in the other eye.

Ophthalmoscopy

1. The features of arteritic papillopathy are the same as those described and illustrated for ischaemic papillopathy (*see* page 61).
2. In 10 per cent of patients, retinal artery occlusion is the presenting feature.

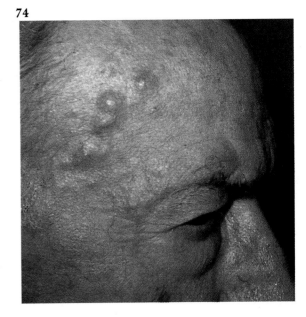

74

74 Giant cell arteritis. The inflamed temporal artery is prominent and nodular; it was tender and non-pulsatile on palpation.

Supplementary findings

Visual acuity is affected in a similar manner to that described for idiopathic ischaemic optic neuropathy (*see* page 62). However, the risk that the second eye will become involved is greater (75 per cent). If treatment is not given immediately after loss of vision in the first eye, blindness in the second eye may follow within a few hours.

Severe cases may show an associated anterior segment ischaemia due to involvement of the choroidal circulation throughout the uveal tract. This may present as iritis, progressing to rubeosis of the iris and neovascular glaucoma.

Associated systemic features

There are many systemic features of giant cell arteritis, which usually precede the onset of arteritic papillopathy. The patient may complain of headache, chiefly involving the temporal and occipital regions. The temporal arteries are thickened and often non-pulsatile (Fig. **74**); severe involvement of the occipital arteries may lead to tenderness and even necrosis of the scalp. Pains in the jaw muscles may be experienced on chewing (jaw claudication). Polymyalgia rheumatica is a common feature, as is weight loss and a feeling of malaise.

Histological confirmation of the disease may be obtained by means of a temporal artery biopsy. An estimation of the erythrocyte sedimentation rate (ESR) should also be carried out, as it is invariably raised. The ESR can therefore be used both to aid diagnosis and to monitor the patient's response to treatment.

Differential diagnosis

Arteritic papillopathy (giant cell arteritis), and the secondary optic atrophy that follows, have to be differentiated from other conditions in which the optic disc is pale and swollen.

Diabetic papillopathy

Juvenile-onset diabetics may develop diabetic papillopathy in the second or third decade of life. The changes that occur involve principally the optic disc and are thought to represent a form of ischaemic papillopathy. The condition occurs bilaterally in the majority of cases. It is important to distinguish between diabetic papillopathy, an example of pseudopapilloedema, and true papilloedema (brought about by raised intracranial pressure) in order to save the patient from unnecessary neurological investigations.

Ophthalmoscopy

The clinical features vary in severity:

1. The optic disc may be hyperaemic and swollen and the margin indistinct; there may be mild oedema in the adjacent retina.
2. In severe cases (Fig. **75**) the findings are similar to those of classic papilloedema (*see* page 75).
3. Diabetic retinopathy, when present, is limited in extent.

75

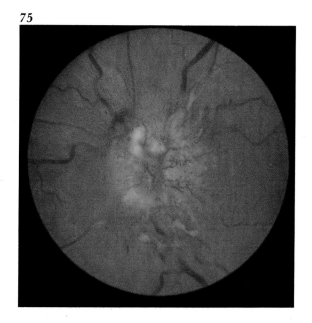

75 Diabetic papillopathy (pseudopapilloedema).

Supplementary findings

Visual loss ranges from mild to moderate in degree and may be transient; it usually recovers spontaneously within 6 months of the onset of symptoms. This is in marked contrast to the severe visual loss typical of the ischaemic optic neuropathies that affect older people (*see* pages, 61, 62). However, the swelling of the optic disc that occurs in diabetic papillopathy may take up to 1 year to resolve and may result in mild secondary optic atrophy. There is no correlation between the changes seen ophthalmoscopically and the eventual visual outcome.

Associated systemic features

The systemic associations are those of diabetes mellitus.

Differential diagnosis

Diabetic papillopathy has to be distinguished:

1. From papilloedema, and from other conditions in which the optic disc is hyperaemic and swollen.
2. From the severe peripapillary retinal oedema brought about by intraretinal leakage in diabetic retinopathy.

The mild secondary optic atrophy that may be associated with diabetic papillopathy has to be distinguished from other conditions in which the optic disc is pale and swollen.

Leber's hereditary optic neuropathy

This hereditary disorder, of unknown aetiology, is difficult to classify. It shows features suggesting that it may be a form of optic neuritis (namely a papillitis), but there is also evidence of vasculopathy. The vascular abnormalities, which are found in relation to the optic disc, may precede the onset of visual symptoms by several months. Progression to optic atrophy and severe visual impairment occurs within about 2 years of onset.

The condition is almost exclusively a disease of young males, usually presenting in the second or third decades of life (although an age range from 5 to 65 years has been reported). The mode of transmission of the disorder has yet to be defined, although the possibility of a mitochondrial mechanism has been suggested. In this inheritance pattern, males do not transmit the disease to their offspring (the mitochondria in the fertilizing spermatozoon are shed as the ovum is penetrated). However, all female carriers transmit the affected mitochondrial DNA (cytoplasmic genetic material) to their male offspring, and to their daughters who may become carriers. It is therefore important that the members of affected families should receive genetic counselling.

Ophthalmoscopy

In the acute stage (Fig. **76**) there is a classic triad of features, two of which are visible on ophthalmoscopy:

1. The optic disc is swollen and hyperaemic.
2. There are dilated, telangiectatic capillaries mainly on, and extending from, the temporal side of the optic disc.
3. Fundus fluorescein angiography (Fig. **77**) reveals that these telangiectasia do not leak dye (cf. papilloedema, *see* page 78).

In the chronic stage secondary optic atrophy occurs (Fig. **78**) and there is a marked reduction in the vascularity associated with the optic disc.

Supplementary findings

As in acute optic neuritis, there is a sudden loss of vision in one eye which may be followed, weeks or months later, by a similar loss of vision in the fellow eye. In Leber's optic

76

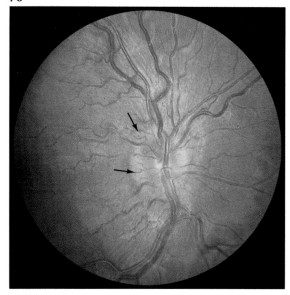

76 Leber's hereditary optic neuropathy (acute stage). The optic disc is hyperaemic and swollen and has dilated capillaries (arrows), mainly on its temporal surface.

78

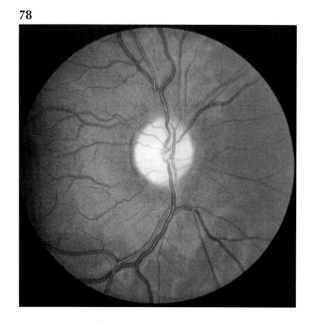

78 Leber's hereditary optic neuropathy (chronic stage). The disc is atrophic and its vascularity is reduced.

77

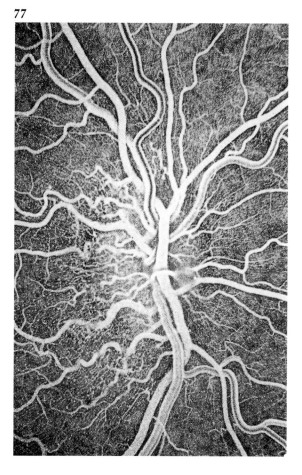

77 Fundus fluorescein angiogram of the case illustrated in Fig. **76**, showing that the abnormal capillaries on the optic disc do not leak dye.

neuropathy, however, this loss of vision is permanent (cf. optic neuritis caused by demyelination; *see* page 59).

The visual field abnormality is typically a centrocaecal defect which parallels the development of optic atrophy.

Associated systemic features

Individuals with this disorder are usually healthy; however, cases with cardiac conduction abnormalities have been reported.

Differential diagnosis

Leber's hereditary optic neuropathy has to be distinguished from other conditions in which:

1. The optic disc is hyperaemic and swollen.
2. There is secondary optic atrophy.

5: Atrophic Abnormalities

Optic atrophy

There are three types of optic atrophy—primary, secondary and consecutive—which may originate as congenital or acquired disorders. All forms of optic atrophy are a consequence of pathological changes occurring at some point along the optic nerve fibres in their passage from the ganglion cells of the retina to the lateral geniculate bodies in the brain. The three types of atrophy present with pallor of the optic disc and reduced visual acuity.

Primary optic atrophy

Both congenital and acquired disorders are included in this category and present with a pale, flat optic disc.

The congenital primary optic atrophies are rare. They may occur as isolated ocular findings which are inherited either in an autosomal dominant or autosomal recessive pattern. The dominant type usually presents between the ages of 5 and 8 years, and visual acuity is only moderately affected. The recessive type presents at an earlier age, with severe visual impairment. Alternatively, congenital primary optic atrophy may be associated with systemic syndromes as, for example, in Friedreich's ataxia. In this condition optic atrophy is associated with cerebellar degeneration.

Acquired primary optic atrophy arises when the retrobulbar portion of the optic nerve is affected following *retrobulbar neuritis* or *retrobulbar neuropathy* (*see* pages 59, 61).

Ophthalmoscopy

1. The optic disc is pale with a clearly defined margin. The pallor generally involves all of the disc, but is often more pronounced on the temporal side (Fig. **79**).
2. The neural rim has atrophied, resulting in loss of the physiological cup and flattening of the disc.

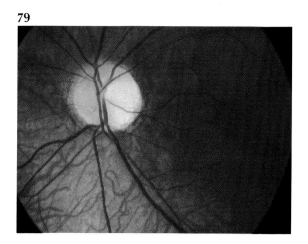

79

79 Primary optic atrophy. The disc is flat and has a well-defined margin; pallor is more pronounced on its temporal side.

Supplementary findings

Visual acuity is affected to a variable degree, depending on the aetiology. Disturbances of colour vision and visual field abnormalities also relate to the primary disorder. In children with severe visual impairment, nystagmus is a common finding.

Associated systemic features

When present, these relate to the underlying disease.

Differential diagnosis

Primary optic atrophy has to be distinguished from:

1. Secondary and consecutive optic atrophy.
2. Those other conditions in which the optic disc is pale and flat.

Secondary optic atrophy

Secondary optic atrophy follows long-standing swelling of the optic disc. Aetiological factors include *papillitis*, the *ischaemic papillopathies* and *papilloedema* (*see* pages 59, 61, 75).

Ophthalmoscopy

The optic disc is pale and swollen; the physiological cup may be partially or completely filled in and the disc margin is poorly defined (*see* Figs. **73B** and **94**).

Consecutive optic atrophy

Consecutive optic atrophy is associated with degenerative changes in the retina. The optic disc is pale and flat, as in primary optic atrophy, but associated retinal and retinal

Supplementary findings

These are linked with the underlying cause of the optic atrophy.

Associated systemic features

When present, these relate to the underlying disorder.

Differential diagnosis

Secondary optic atrophy has to be distinguished from:

1. Primary and consecutive optic atrophy.
2. Those other conditions in which the optic disc is pale and swollen.

vascular changes indicate the origin of the pathological process. *Retinitis pigmentosa*, described in this section, is the prime example of a retinal disorder leading to consecutive

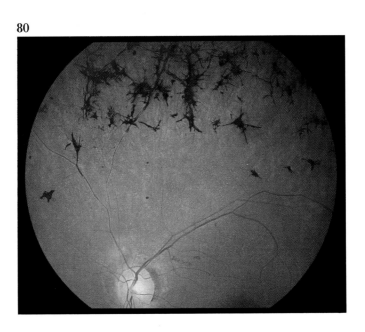

80

80 Retinitis pigmentosa with 'bone spicule' pigmentation in the peripheral retina, overlying the retinal vessels. The optic disc is atrophic, and the retinal vessels are attenuated.

optic atrophy. It is an inherited condition, transmitted in a variety of hereditary patterns. Retinitis pigmentosa and its associated optic atrophy may present as an independent ocular disorder, or be accompanied by other ocular abnormalities; alternatively the ocular changes may form part of a syndrome with an underlying metabolic disorder.

Ophthalmoscopy

In consecutive optic atrophy linked with retinitis pigmentosa (Fig. **80**):

1. The optic disc has a waxy pallor; it is flat and its margin is well defined.
2. The central retinal vessels are attenuated.
3. There are scattered areas of pigmentary degeneration in the peripheral fundus, showing a characteristic 'bone corpuscle' configuration and overlying the retinal vessels. This pathognomic abnormality may be missed unless the pupil is dilated and the peripheral retina examined.

Supplementary findings

The visual acuity is variably affected, depending on the region and extent of retinal involvement. A ring scotoma often occurs. Most commonly, peripheral vision is progressively affected and central vision is retained until late; the latter declines, however, as the scotoma encroaches upon the macula. Typical symptoms of retinitis pigmentosa are night blindness and problems with dark adaptation.

Other ocular abnormalities include posterior subcapsular cataract, chronic open-angle glaucoma and myopia.

Associated systemic features

Several syndromes have been described, although in some the metabolic defect remains to be identified. A well-known example is the Laurence–Moon–Biedl syndrome, in which retinitis pigmentosa is associated with obesity, mental retardation, polydactyli and hypogonadism.

Differential diagnosis

Consecutive optic atrophy has to be distinguished from:

1. Primary and secondary optic atrophy.
2. Those other conditions in which the optic disc is pale and flat.

Other atrophic conditions

Myopia

There are three types of myopia, of which axial myopia is the most serious; it is thought to be caused by a genetically determined developmental defect. In the other two types, namely curvature myopia and index myopia, particular characteristics of different components of the eye affect refraction.

Axial myopia is characterized by an increase in the anteroposterior diameter of the eye, with secondary degenerative changes affecting the whole of the posterior segment. There are two forms of this condition:

1. *Simple myopia*, in which the eye is larger than normal but remains healthy.
2. *Pathological* or *progressive myopia*, in which the eye increases in size up to the third or fourth decade of life and continuing retinal degeneration results in severe visual impairment.

Ophthalmoscopy (Figs. 81–84)

Examination of the patient's eye often proves difficult because of the refractive error, and it may be helpful to examine the fundus with the patient's own spectacles in place.

1. The optic disc is sometimes distorted; it may also be tilted owing to oblique insertion of the optic nerve head into the globe. The tilt is usually in a lateral direction (cf. tilted disc syndrome, *see* page 24). Tilting of the disc causes the retinal blood vessels to enter and exit from the disc at atypical angles and appear dragged; the nasal vessels curve around the elevated nasal sector of the disc and the temporal vessels pursue a straightened course, often traversing a myopic crescent.
2. The myopic crescent is a pale area, usually lying temporal to the optic disc, although it sometimes has an annular configuration and completely encircles the disc, making it appear spuriously large. The crescent or annulus represents an area of pale sclera, visible because the overlying retinal pigment epithelium and choroid fail to

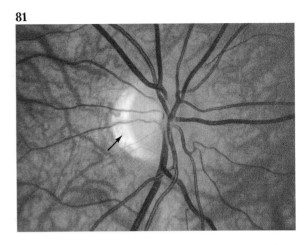

81

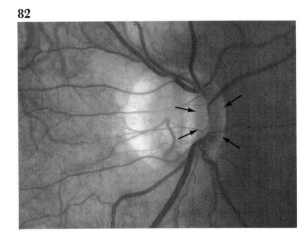

82

81 Myopia. There is a white scleral crescent (arrow) on the temporal side of the optic disc.

82 Lateral tilting of the optic disc in myopia. The disc (arrows) is seen 'edge on' and appears spuriously small; the temporal retinal vessels pass horizontally over a large, pale scleral crescent.

reach the disc margin. The outer border of the crescent or annulus may be pigmented.

3. The retina surrounding the optic disc may be thinned and show white lines of atrophy (lacquer cracks) which are breaks in Bruch's membrane.
4. A Foster–Fuchs' spot is sometimes present at the macula (*see* below).
5. The peripheral retina may be atrophic, with holes or tears, predisposing to retinal detachment.
6. A posterior staphyloma may develop in severe cases, when retinal vessels are seen to dip into the cavity produced by the herniation.

Supplementary findings

Distance vision is affected and requires correction by lenses. Colour vision, particularly blue/yellow discrimination, is sometimes abnormal and dark adaptation may be affected in cases where the peripheral retina is involved. The vitreous is abnormal, causing patients to complain of seeing 'floaters'.

In severe myopia, central vision may slowly deteriorate as a result of atrophic changes localized in the macula. In addition, subretinal neovascularization and haemorrhage in this area may cause sudden loss of central vision; subsequent pigmentary scar formation gives rise to a Foster–Fuchs' spot.

Retinal degeneration, particularly at the periphery, predisposes to retinal detachment. Herniation of the posterior wall of the globe may occur in cases of progressive myopia, forming a staphyloma. This rare complication has a severe effect on vision.

Should glaucoma develop in myopic patients, it is difficult to monitor. This is because abnormalities of the optic disc, reduced visual acuity and changes in the peripheral field are common to both conditions.

Associated systemic features

None known.

83

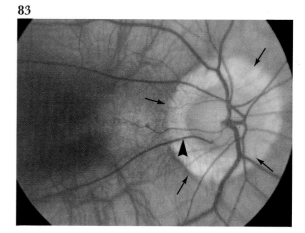

84

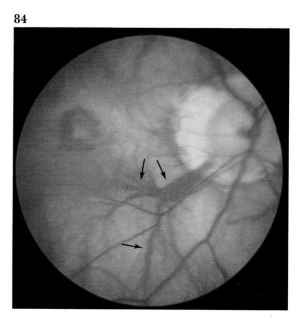

83 A scleral annulus (arrows) surrounds the optic disc, making it appear spuriously large. The cilioretinal artery (triangle) is an incidental finding.

84 Severe myopia with a pigmented Foster–Fuchs' spot at the macula. Major choroidal vessels (arrows) are visible through the atrophic retina. A scleral annulus is also present. (The fundus details are out of focus owing to the high refractive error.)

Differential diagnosis

Myopia has to be differentiated from those other conditions in which:

1. The optic disc appears enlarged, or
2. Excavated.
3. There is peripapillary pigmentary change.
4. Retinal vessels appear dragged.

Glaucoma

Evaluation of the appearance of the optic disc plays a key role in both the diagnosis and management of patients with glaucoma. A sustained rise in intraocular pressure is associated with damage to the fibres of the optic nerve as they pass over the rim of the optic disc. The resultant atrophy of nerve tissue causes narrowing of the neural rim of the optic disc, correlated with an increase in the size of the physiological cup. This sign—known as cupping of the optic disc—is the hallmark of glaucoma.

The size of the physiological cup is expressed in terms of the ratio, vertical dimension of cup:vertical diameter of optic disc. While these dimensions show a wide variation in normal eyes (*see* page 12), a cup:disc ratio of more than 0.6 is suggestive of glaucomatous cupping. Furthermore, since the two optic discs are normally cupped symmetrically, asymmetry in cup size should also alert to the possibility of glaucoma. Other characteristic abnormalities in the structure of the optic disc are described below.

Ophthalmoscopy
(Figs. **85**, **86**)

1. The optic disc has a pathologically enlarged cup, which may become deep enough to expose the cribriform plate at its base. The enlarged cup is pale and the cribriform plate has a grey, sieve-like appearance.
2. The neural rim of the optic disc becomes narrowed and may show a sector of pallor, most commonly situated in its inferotemporal quadrant. This represents an area of nerve fibre atrophy which may extend into the adjacent retina where it takes the form of a radial groove or split. This is dark in appearance and is best seen using the red-free (green) filter on the ophthalmoscope.
3. The central retinal vessels emerge in a hook-like fashion, curving upwards from beneath the undermined neural rim of the disc.
4. Splinter haemorrhages, indicative of active neural degeneration, may be present on the neural rim of the optic disc, most commonly in the inferotemporal quadrant.

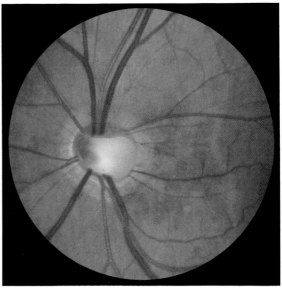

85

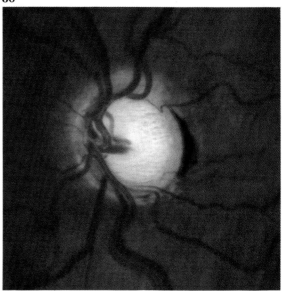

86

85 Glaucomatous cupping of the optic disc. The central retinal vessels emerge in a hook-like fashion from beneath the neural rim of the disc. At their origin, in the base of the deepened cup, the vessels lie behind the plane of focus.

86 Glaucoma. The sieve-like cribriform plate is visible in the base of the enlarged cup which occupies nearly all of the disc area. The cup:disc ratio is about 0.8 and the neural rim is attenuated. The crescent of dark pigment around the temporal side of the optic disc is a normal variant and unrelated to the glaucoma.

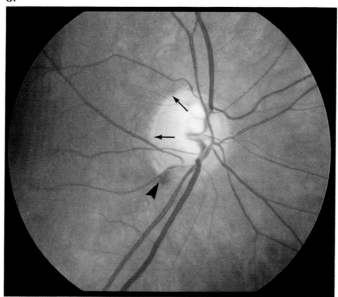

87 Advanced glaucoma. The neural rim (arrows) on the temporal side of the optic disc is extremely attenuated and the retinal vessels are displaced nasally. The pale disc appears spuriously flat. A splinter haemorrhage (triangle) on the inferotemporal quadrant of the neural rim is a classic finding.

5. In end-stage glaucoma (Fig. **87**) the atrophic neural rim may be narrowed to such an extent that the enlarged, pale cup occupies almost the total area of the optic disc. Absence of normal disc tissue around an extensive central area of pallor may lead the inexperienced observer to conclude that the physiological cup is absent and the disc is flat and pale. Thus advanced glaucoma may be misinterpreted as primary optic atrophy.

Supplementary findings

The main feature of glaucoma is a progressive constriction of the peripheral field, but this takes place so slowly that patients are usually unaware of the change. This insidious development makes early diagnosis difficult, for visual acuity may remain normal, even when the sight is reduced to 'tunnel vision'.

Associated systemic features

There are no specific systemic associations.

Differential diagnosis

Glaucoma has to be distinguished from other conditions in which the optic disc is excavated.

Avulsion

Avulsion—a forcible separation of the optic nerve from the posterior aspect of the globe—occurs as a result of severe trauma to the eye or orbital region. It causes blindness. Following the acute stage, the posterior pole of the fundus undergoes atrophic changes which may mimic congenital or other acquired abnormalities involving the optic disc.

Ophthalmoscopy

In the acute phase (Fig. **88**):

The structure of the posterior pole of the fundus is disrupted; the optic disc is difficult to identify and numerous haemorrhages are present in the peripapillary retina. In addition, the view of the fundus may be obscured by haemorrhage, either in the vitreous, or in the anterior segment of the eye.

At later stages (Fig. **89**):

1. The tissues that comprise the normal optic disc disappear and are replaced by a deep, funnel-like depression. Those retinal blood vessels that remain intact curve over the edge of the funnel.
2. The circumpapillary retina and choroid undergo atrophy, with accompanying pigmentary scar formation.

Supplementary findings

The affected eye is blind and the afferent pupillary reflex is absent. In the acute phase there is likely to be evidence of trauma to the eye or orbital region.

Differential diagnosis

Avulsion of the optic disc has to be distinguished from other conditions in which the optic disc appears excavated.

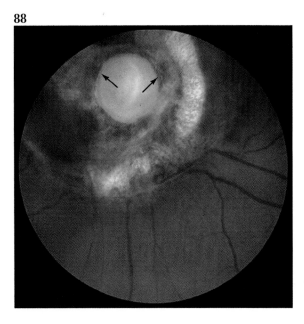

88 **Avulsion of the optic disc, acute stage.** The optic nerve head has herniated posteriorly to reveal the scleral canal (arrows). The retinal vessels and retina are torn and there is a large haemorrhage on the margin of the herniation.

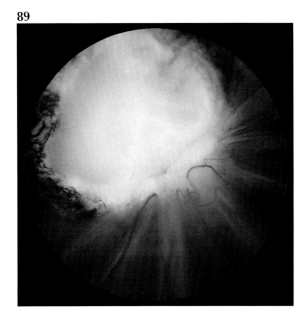

89 **Later phase** (case illustrated in Fig. 88). A large, pale, funnel-like excavation can be seen at the site previously occupied by the optic nerve head. The appearance mimics that of an optic disc coloboma.

6: Papilloedema and pseudopapilloedema

Papilloedema is swelling of the optic nerve head caused by raised intracranial pressure; thus it invariably signifies serious underlying pathology, requiring urgent investigation. In order to avoid subjecting the patient to unnecessary neurological investigation, however, true papilloedema has to be distinguished from papilloedema associated with accelerated hypertension, and from cases of 'pseudopapilloedema' in which the optic disc similarly appears hyperaemic and swollen. The latter conditions include optic disc drusen and hypermetropia, as well as diabetic papillopathy (*see* page 63).

Papilloedema

Swelling of the optic nerve head in papilloedema is thought to be caused by a disturbance of axoplasmic flow in the optic nerve fibres, secondary to raised intracranial pressure. Papilloedema is a non-specific, non-localizing sign of raised intracranial pressure: it gives no indication of either the nature or the site of the primary disorder, hence its presence is an indication for urgent referral and neurological investigation.

Factors responsible for raised intracranial pressure include space-occupying lesions in the brain, such as a tumour or haemorrhage, the long-term use of certain drugs, for example, systemic steroids or the contraceptive pill, tetracycline, or vitamin A; also exposure to poisons, such as lead.

Papilloedema almost always occurs bilaterally. However, a tumour of the frontal lobe may give rise to the Foster–Kennedy syndrome (*see also* page 62). In this syndrome the optic disc of one eye presents with atrophy due to direct pressure of the tumour on the optic nerve, whereas the disc in the fellow eye shows papilloedema caused by raised intracranial pressure.

Ophthalmoscopy

The appearance of the optic disc and fundus differ in the early, acute, long-standing and atrophic phases of papilloedema (Figs. **90–92**, **94**).

In the early phase:

1. The optic disc is swollen and has an indistinct margin. Because of the variation in the relative density of nerve fibres in the neural rim, swelling (brought about by the accumulation of axoplasm) is first seen in the nasal quadrant of the disc and then in its superior and inferior sectors.
2. The physiological cup is maintained, giving the disc a cylindrical appearance.
3. The disc is hyperaemic due to dilatation of the capillaries.
4. The retinal veins, which may be congested, are invariably non-pulsatile.
5. A circumpapillary accumulation of fluid may result in concentric retinal folds (Paton's folds and choroidal folds. These changes are best seen with the red-free (green) filter of the ophthalmoscope.

In the acute phase:

1. The optic disc becomes increasingly swollen and elevated; however, the physiological cup may still be maintained.
2. Retinal venous congestion becomes more pronounced; some of the blood vessels may be partially obscured at the edge of the disc, as they dip over and curve beneath its raised outer margin.

90   Early papilloedema. The disc is hyperaemic and the inferonasal margin (arrows) indistinct.

91   Acute papilloedema with florid swelling of the optic disc. Hyperaemia is present, brought about by dilatation of the capillaries and congestion of the veins. Axoplasmic debris forms pale accumulations on the elevated rim of the disc. The swollen neural rim and still definable physiological cup give the optic disc a cylindrical appearance.

90

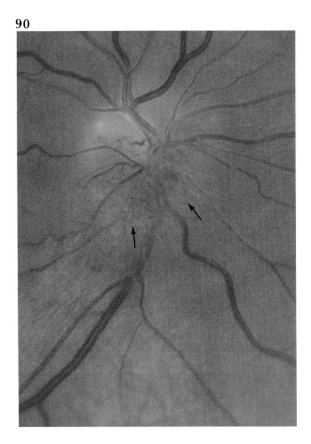

91

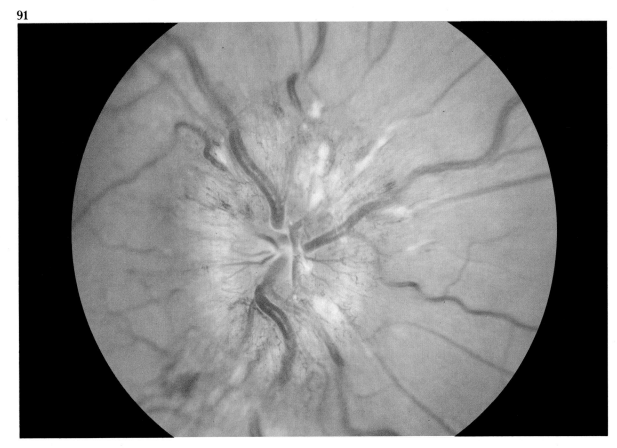

92 Paton's folds (arrows) in acute papilloedema, as viewed with the red-free (green) filter of the ophthalmoscope.

92

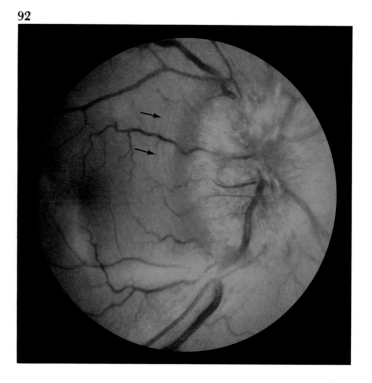

93A

93B

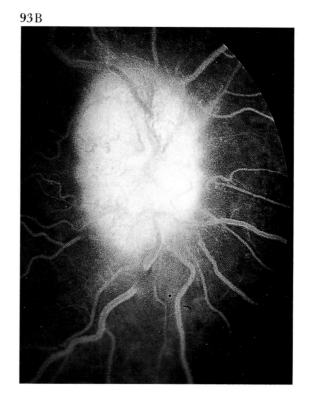

93 Fundus fluorescein angiogram of papill-oedema. (**A**) Capillaries on the optic disc are dilated and (**B**) subsequently leak dye profusely.

3. Numerous flame-shaped haemorrhages are seen on the disc margin, with associated accumulations of axoplasmic debris.
4. Fluid and exudates may accumulate in the retina and a macular star may develop, most prominent on the nasal aspect of the macula.

In the long-standing phase:

1. The disc is markedly swollen and the physiological cup is obliterated, giving the classical 'champagne cork' appearance.
2. Circulatory adjustments result in the resolution of venous congestion and retinal oedema.

In the atrophic stage:

1. The swollen optic disc becomes pale owing to secondary optic atrophy (*see* page 68). Neuronal degenerative changes may produce punctate white opacities in the superficial nerve fibre layer (cf. optic disc drusen, *see* page 81).
2. The retinal arteries are often attenuated.
3. There may be circumpapillary choroidal pallor and atrophy of the retinal pigment epithelium, with areas of pigmentary clumping.

Supplementary findings

Visual symptoms are rarely a presenting feature in the early stages of papilloedema. Later, however, transient obscurations of vision may occur; these are especially likely during manoeuvres such as coughing or straining which increase intracranial pressure. In the atrophic stage, visual acuity may be variably affected and colour vision is usually abnormal.

The visual field typically shows an enlarged blind spot (cf. the central scotoma in papillitis, *see* page 59). Peripheral field constriction only occurs when secondary optic atrophy supervenes.

Double vision may be caused by involvement of the 6th cranial nerve and resultant paralysis of the lateral rectus muscle. This is another non-localizing sign of raised intracranial pressure; it arises when the meninges are stretched, exerting tension on the 6th nerve as it passes over the superior ridge of the petrous part of the temporal bone.

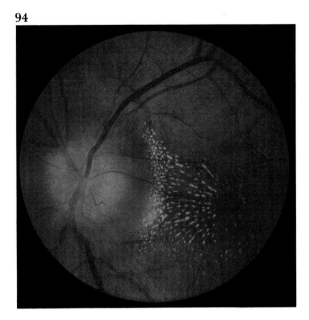

94 **Papilloedema** with a macular star, more prominent on the nasal side of the macula. The optic disc is beginning to show secondary optic atrophy.

Fundus fluorescein angiography shows that in papilloedema the optic disc capillaries are dilated and leak dye profusely (*see* Fig. **93**). This feature helps to distinguish papilloedema from pseudopapilloedema, but not from papillitis—in which the capillaries also leak dye.

Associated systemic features

Associated systemic features are those directly related to raised intracranial pressure and include headache and vomiting (without nausea), typically worse on waking and exacerbated by straining. Other features are those related to the underlying aetiology.

Differential diagnosis

1. Papilloedema has to be differentiated from other conditions in which the optic disc is hyperaemic and swollen.
2. When secondary optic atrophy follows, it has to be distinguished from other conditions in which the optic disc is pale and swollen.

Hypertension

The rate of progression and severity of systemic hypertension may be reflected by changes in the retinal blood vessels which can be directly observed ophthalmoscopically. In mild and moderate hypertension, retinal aterioles show a reduction in calibre and there is 'nipping' of the venules at arteriovenous crossings. Accelerated hypertension is associated with more widespread arteriolar constriction and various manifestations of retinal ischaemia, as well as papilloedema.

Papilloedema associated with hypertension requires differentiation from that brought about by raised intracranial pressure secondary to a space-occupying lesion. In addition, the characteristic, bilateral, retinovascular changes may be a presenting feature of hypertension and signal the need for prompt treatment of the systemic disorder. The classification of hypertensive retinopathy into various grades of severity has been used as a prognostic aid in the management of patients.

Ophthalmoscopy

The ophthalmoscopic features are related to the stage of progression and severity of the hypertension: hypertensive retinopathy is traditionally divided into four grades.

In Grade 1:

The retinal vessels are slightly narrowed and there is mild 'nipping' of the venules at arteriovenous crossings.

In Grade 2 (Fig. 95):

1. Changes at the arteriovenous crossings are more pronounced and the retinal arterioles show focal attenuation.
2. The burnishing arteriolar light reflexes, known as 'copper-' and 'silver-wiring' (*see* page 14) are increased out of proportion in relation to the age of the patient.

In Grade 3:

The features are as described for Grade 2 but, in addition, there are superficial, splinter haemorrhages in the nerve fibre layer. Cotton-wool infarcts, reflecting retinal ischaemia, are randomly scattered throughout the posterior pole of the fundus (cf. papilloedema, *see* page 75).

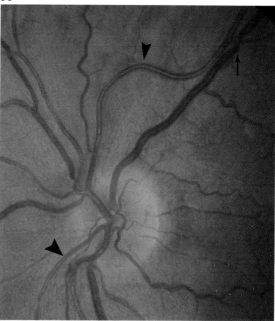

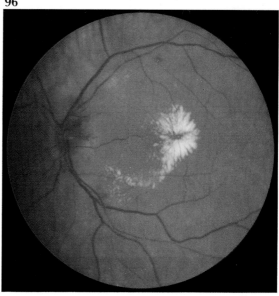

95 Early hypertensive retinopathy with arteriovenous 'nipping' (arrow). The retinal arterioles show focal narrowing and an increased light reflex —'copper-wiring' (triangles).

96 Accelerated hypertension with papilloedema and a macular star.

In Grade 4 (accelerated hypertension) (Figs. **96, 97**):

1. The features are as described for Grade 3, with the addition of papilloedema.
2. Retinal oedema is present and hard exudates may collect around the fovea, producing a typical macular star.

3. There may be ischaemic choroidal infarcts appearing as pale, round or wedge-shaped areas in the peripheral retina (Elschnig's spots, Siegrist's streaks).

Supplementary findings

Visual acuity is usually normal although, in severe hypertension, transient obscurations of vision sometimes occur; these are typically altitudinal. Sustained accelerated hypertension may result in progressive and permanent loss of vision. Acute-onset hypertension, as in pregnancy (eclampsia), occasionally gives rise to bilateral exudative retinal detachments; these resolve with control of the blood pressure but may leave residual mottling in the retinal pigment epithelium.

The pupillary reaction is usually normal, helping to distinguish hypertension from ischaemic optic neuropathy in which there is a severe decrease in visual acuity. However, it is

noteworthy that hypertension is sometimes involved in the aetiology of ischaemic optic neuropathy. Similarly, hypertension can play a role in the aetiology of retinal vascular occlusions.

Associated systemic features

These relate to cardiac, renal or cerebral complications of the disorder.

Differential diagnosis

1. Papilloedema due to accelerated hypertension must be differentiated from other conditions in which the optic disc is hyperaemic and swollen.
2. The signs of retinal ischaemia in severe hypertension have to be distinguished from those occurring in central retinal vascular occlusion (*see* pages 49, 51) and in diabetic retinopathy (*see* page 54).

97

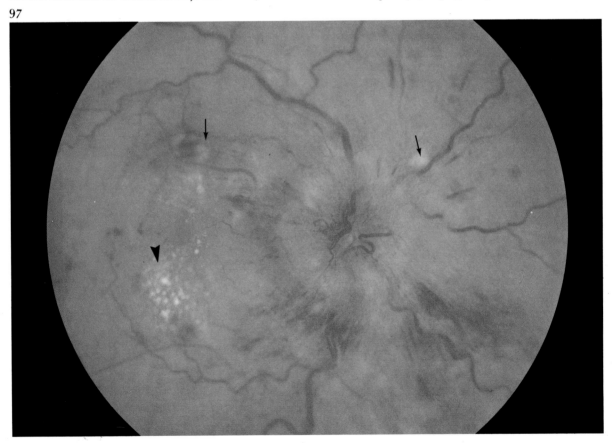

97 Accelerated hypertension with cotton-wool infarcts (arrows) and retinal haemorrhages widely scattered through the posterior pole of the fundus.

An early macular star is also present (triangle); (cf. Fig. **91** showing 'florid' papilloedema).

Optic disc drusen

Drusen derives from the German word meaning gland, or gland-like swelling. Optic disc drusen are manifestations of a congenital abnormality in which deposits accumulate in the optic nerve head. A causative factor is thought to be a reduction in the size of the lamina cribrosa (*see* page 19) which inhibits the process of axonal flow in the nerve fibres and predisposes to axonal degeneration. Accumulation of debris (chiefly calcified mitochondrial material) anterior to the cribriform plate leads to swelling of the optic nerve head.

Although this is a congenital abnormality, the drusen generally remain 'buried' during childhood and only become apparent during the teenage years, when they present as single or multiple swellings of the optic disc.

Drusen occur almost exclusively in white races, about 1 per cent of the population being affected. The drusen generally occur bilaterally (70 per cent) and the condition is transmitted as an irregular dominant trait with incomplete penetrance. Examination of older members of the family may therefore help to confirm a suspected diagnosis in a child.

Optic disc drusen should not be confused with retinal drusen which form part of the condition known as age-related macular degeneration. Retinal drusen (*see* Fig. **104**) consist of hyaline material which accumulates as a result of incomplete metabolism of degenerating rods and cones by the retinal pigment epithelium. These drusen form rounded elevations on Bruch's membrane, which displace the overlying retinal pigment epithelium and neural retina.

Ophthalmoscopy

In children (Fig. **98**):

1. The optic disc is small and pink and the drusen are 'hidden' within the substance of the nerve head.
2. Often the margin of the disc is indistinct, giving the appearance of pseudopapilloedema.
3. The central retinal vessels may show anomalous branching (10 per cent of cases); cilioretinal arteries commonly occur (*see* page 43).

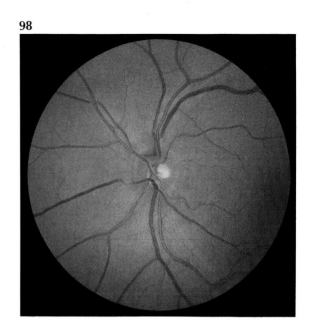

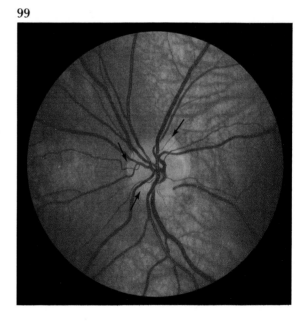

98 Optic disc drusen in a child. The disc is small and appears hyperaemic, owing to 'buried' drusen.

99 Optic disc drusen in an adolescent. The disc, although small, shows several drusen (arrows) which give the margin an irregular outline. A cilioretinal artery is present.

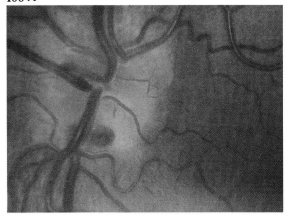

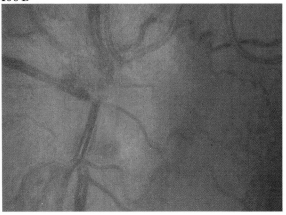

4. The retinal veins are not distended and spontaneous retinal pulsation is not affected (cf. early papilloedema, *see* page 75).

In adolescents and adults (Figs. **99–101, 104**):

1. Drusen are seen as single or multiple glistening, semi-translucent swellings which may coalesce and give the disc a yellow-pink appearance.
2. The optic disc may become enlarged and its border indistinct or irregular.
3. The physiological cup is obliterated (cf. papilloedema, *see* page 75).
4. There may be splinter haemorrhages on the disc surface and subretinal haemorrhages in the peripapillary area.

Supplementary findings

Optic disc drusen are usually asymptomatic. However, progressive compression of the nerve fibres may lead to variable patterns of visual field defects.

A well-known complication is the development of a juxtapapillary subretinal neovascular membrane. This may lead to haemorrhage and sudden loss of vision (*see* Fig. **103**). Subsequent retinal scar formation is self-limiting, however, and—provided the macula is spared—visual acuity is only moderately affected. Rarely, there is infarction of the optic nerve head and ischaemic papillopathy, leading to severe loss of vision.

Other associated ocular features include retinitis pigmentosa (*see* page 68) and, possibly, angioid streaks in the retina (*see* page 110).

100 Progressive swelling of the optic disc owing to drusen. (**A**) The disc margin, although distorted, is still discernible. (**B**) Two years later: the disc is swollen and ill-defined, mimicking papilloedema. The central retinal vessels show anomalous branching.

Fundus fluorescein angiography plays an important role in differentiating between optic disc drusen and papilloedema. Disc drusen pathognomically show autofluorescence before injection of the dye (*see* Fig. **102**). During the angiogram the drusen are hyperfluorescent but do not leak dye, or only minimally so. Large drusen become calcified and show up on computerized tomography or ultrasonography.

Associated systemic features

None known.

Differential diagnosis

1. In children, optic disc drusen should be differentiated from other conditions in which the optic disc is small.
2. Early disc drusen should be differentiated from papilloedema and from other conditions in which the optic disc appears hyperaemic and swollen.
3. Advanced disc drusen should be differentiated from other conditions in which the optic disc is pale and swollen.

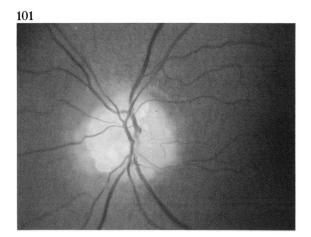

101 Advanced optic disc drusen.

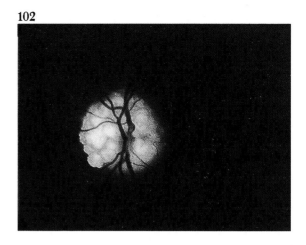

102 Autofluorescence of the disc drusen shown in Fig. **101**.

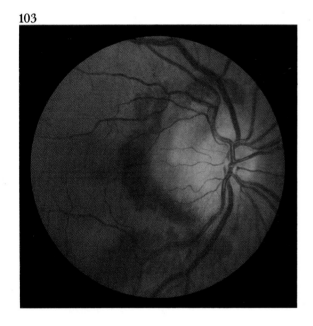

103 Circumpapillary haemorrhage associated with optic disc drusen.

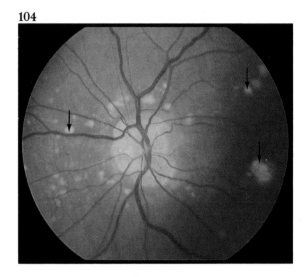

104 Retinal drusen (arrows) presenting as an incidental finding in this case of optic disc drusen. Retinal drusen, an age-related abnormality, should not be confused with optic disc drusen.

Hypermetropia

In this congenital abnormality the eye has a shorter axial length than normal. The hypermetropic eye also has a small optic disc which appears hyperaemic and spuriously swollen, because of diminution of the physiological cup. These features bear a superficial resemblance to papilloedema; however, many of the features described below aid the differentiation between hypermetropia and papilloedema caused by raised intracranial pressure (*see* page 75).

Ophthalmoscopy

1. The small, pink optic disc appears elevated and congested, but its capillaries are not dilated (Fig. **105**).
2. The central retinal vessels crowd the centre of the small optic disc (Fig. **106**); spontaneous venous pulsation is not affected.
3. In severe cases, horizontal choroidal folds are occasionally found in the peripheral fundus (cf. concentric Paton's folds in papilloedema).

Supplementary findings

Near visual acuity is reduced and the refractive error requires correction with lenses. Because of the small size of the eye the anterior chamber is shallow. In the elderly this predisposes to acute narrow-angle glaucoma as the lens increases in size, particularly when becoming cataractous. During fundus fluorescein angiography, capillaries on the optic disc do not leak dye (cf. papilloedema).

Associated systemic features

None known.

Differential diagnosis

Hypermetropia has to be distinguished from other conditions in which the optic disc appears:

1. Small.
2. Hyperaemic and swollen.

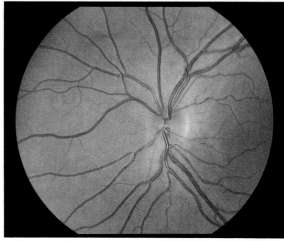

105

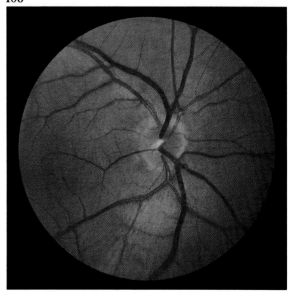

106

105   A hypermetropic optic disc.

106   Central retinal vessels crowd the small, hypermetropic optic disc.

7: Tumours and Tumour-like Conditions

Developmental abnormalities

Melanocytoma

A melanocytoma is a benign, pigmented tumour; it should not be confused with the highly malignant choroidal melanoma (*see* page 101). A melanocytoma arises from dendritic melanocytes. It is a special form of uveal naevus and can occur anywhere in the eye where there are cell rests of primitive uveal melanocytes, for example, in the uveal tract (choroid, ciliary body, iris) and also in the conjunctiva and sclera; it most commonly occurs on the optic disc.

Melanocytomas most frequently arise in the pigmented racial groups and in caucasians of Mediterranean origin (cf. melanoma). It is more frequently seen in females than males; there is no hereditary pattern.

Ophthalmoscopy

1. The tumour varies in colour from grey to jet black. It is often eccentrically placed on the optic disc, extending over the disc margin and covering it to a variable degree. Where it extends into the nerve fibre layer of the retina, the edges of the tumour may appear feathery (Fig. **107**).
2. The optic disc adjacent to the tumour is usually of normal appearance, but may be swollen. The swelling is thought to be caused by disturbances of axonal flow and may extend into the juxtapapillary region.
3. In 50 per cent of cases there is a juxtapapillary choroidal naevus which is contiguous with the melanocytoma on the optic disc. There may also be evidence of degeneration in the retinal pigment epithelium in this region, but there are no juxtapapillary retinal traction lines (cf. combined hamartoma of the retina and RPE, *see* page 90).
4. The calibre and course of the retinal vessels are unaltered (cf. combined hamartoma), although those emerging from the substance of the tumour, or overlying it, may be sheathed.

Supplementary findings

Visual acuity is usually normal; the condition is most often asymptomatic and discovered at routine eye examination. However, in 75 per cent of cases the visual field shows an enlarged blind spot; in 20 per cent there is an arcuate scotoma and in 10 per cent a nasal step.

The tumour is usually stationary but in 15 per cent of patients it slowly increases in size, over a time span of from 5 to 20 years; some visual loss may then occur.

Although malignant transformation with an accelerated growth pattern can take place, this is a rare event. Nevertheless, patients with a melanocytoma should be monitored in the long term, by means of fundus photography, fluorescein angiography and serial vision field testing.

The fluorescein angiogram is pathognomic (Fig. **108**) and provides a method for positively differentiating between a melanocytoma and a melanoma. The pigmented melanocytoma shows hypofluorescence through all phases of the angiogram, in contrast to the highly fluorescent vascular melanoma.

Associated systemic features

None known.

Differential diagnosis

A melanocytoma has to be distinguished from other pigmented swellings on the optic disc.

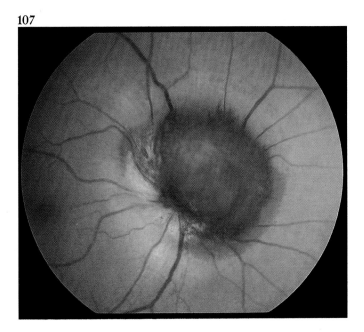

107 Melanocytoma of the optic disc, almost completely obscuring the normal disc tissue and extending into the juxtapapillary region.

108

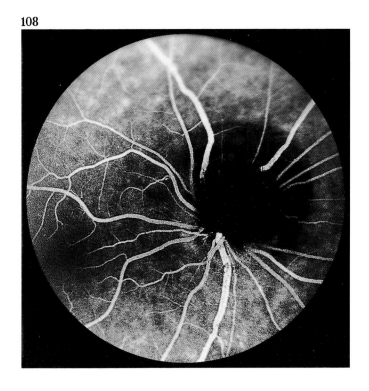

108 Fundus fluorescein angiogram (same patient as in Fig. **107**) demonstrating poor vascular supply and hypofluorescence of the tumour (cf. choroidal melanoma, Fig. **129**).

Hamartomas

Hamartomas are tumour-like malformations which are the outcome of defective maturation within an organ primordium: hyperplasia, or over-development, of one or more of the normal cellular components results in disorganization and malformation of that structure. Thus hamartomas contain tissues normal for the site in which they occur, but arranged in a disorderly or bizarre manner. These congenitally acquired anomalies are non-metastasizing; their growth during postnatal life is correlated with increments in general body size.

Hamartomas of the eye are of three types. The first arises as a result of defective development of supporting elements (astrocytes) of the optic nerve head and retinal nerve fibre layer; the second chiefly involves the retinal pigment epithelium and the third type (of which there are two examples) affects blood vessels of the optic disc and retina.

Astrocytic hamartoma

This developmental disorder rarely occurs as an isolated ocular finding. Its clinical significance lies in the frequent association between astrocytic hamartomas and two of the phakomatoses, namely tuberous sclerosis (Bourneville's disease) and neurofibromatosis (von Recklinghausen's disease).

The hamartoma derives from astrocytes in the optic nerve head and nerve fibre layer of the retina, where it is associated with the ganglion cells. It may involve the optic nerve head alone, and/or may develop in the peripheral retina. Astrocytic hamartomas frequently present bilaterally and more than one may be present in the same eye.

Ophthalmoscopy

1. An astrocytic hamartoma forms a tumour-like mass, usually situated near or on the optic disc; it may also present in the peripheral retina.
2. It may form a semi-translucent mass which is smooth and probably represents an early stage in the development of the hamartoma.
3. The more mature state has a number of striking characteristics, forming a mulberry-like, white reflective mass, which may become calcified (Fig. **109**).

109

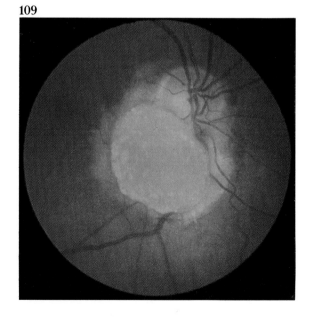

109 Astrocytic hamartoma (mulberry tumour) extending from the optic disc.

4. Astrocytic hamartomas range in size, from the equivalent of approximately half to several diameters of the optic disc.
5. They are very vascular and blood vessels can often be seen coursing through their substance. An area of fibrous proliferation may extend from the hamartoma, distorting the blood vessels.

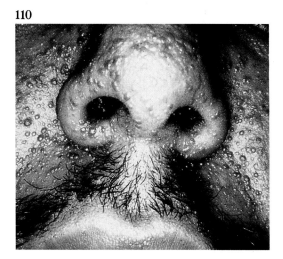

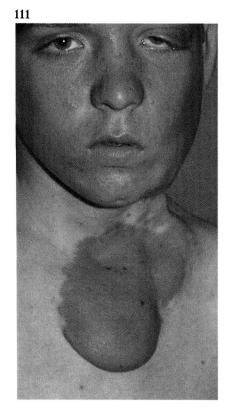

110 Tuberous sclerosis with adenoma sebaceum of the face.

111 Neurofibromatosis. Plexiform neuromas involve the left eyelid, face and trunk.

112

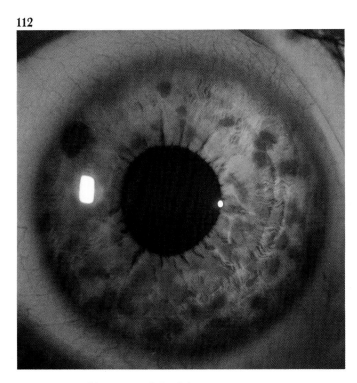

112 Neurofibromas of the iris.

Supplementary findings

Astrocytic hamartomas are often an incidental finding on routine eye examination. Their growth rate rarely exceeds that of surrounding structures, but if they enlarge sufficiently to compress the optic disc they may lead to visual field defects. Rarely they may bleed, causing vitreous haemorrhage.

Fundus fluorescein angiography assists their diagnosis. Prior to injection of the dye, astrocytic hamartomas may exhibit autofluorescence; however, the subsequent angiogram confirms the presence of a vascular component (cf. optic disc drusen, *see* page 81).

Associated ocular and systemic features

As already indicated, there are important associations with tuberous sclerosis and neurofibromatosis. Both of these conditions are transmitted as autosomal dominant traits.

Tuberous sclerosis (Fig. **110**) *(Bourneville's disease)* is characterized by the classic triad of adenoma sebaceum (angiofibromas of the face), mental deficiency and epilepsy; hamartomas arise in the brain. An ocular astrocytic hamartoma occurs in about 50 per cent of cases with tuberous sclerosis. It is an early sign and may assist diagnosis of the syndrome.

In *neurofibromatosis von Recklinghausen's disease)* pigmented skin lesions ('café-au-lait spots') and multiple neurofibromas are usually prominent (Fig. **111**). Plexiform neuromas in the skin may give rise to an 'elephant-man' appearance; these neuromas may be accompanied by other tumours, all of which arise in tissues derived from embryonic ectoderm and result in numerous ocular and systemic manifestations.

Ocular manifestations include the following:

1. Orbital and eyelid abnormalities: proptosis caused by optic nerve tumours; plexiform neuroma of the eyelid; lagophthalmos caused by acoustic neuroma.
2. Abnormalities of the globe: corneal anaesthesia (trigeminal neuroma); plexiform neuroma of the conjunctiva; neurofibroma of the iris (Fig. **112**); buphthalmos.
3. Fundus abnormalities: papilloedema and optic atrophy; myelination of the optic disc.

Differential diagnosis

Astrocytic hamartomas have to be differentiated from other conditions in which the optic disc is pale, swollen and distorted.

Combined hamartoma of the retina and retinal pigment epithelium

Originally named a retinal pigment epithelium hamartoma, this abnormality is now thought to affect additional retinal elements and is known as a combined hamartoma of the retina and retinal pigment epithelium (RPE). The current theory is that changes in the RPE are secondary to a deep intraretinal vascular hamartoma. Thus the area of pigmentary disturbance shows an apparent increase in the number of associated retinal vessels, which are dilated and tortuous; superficially there is a thickened epiretinal membrane.

The combined hamartoma may affect the optic disc, or occur as an isolated finding in the retina. The defect usually occurs unilaterally. There is no described hereditary pattern.

Ophthalmoscopy

1. Characteristically there is a charcoal-grey pigmented abnormality at least partially overlying the optic disc; its feathery border extends into the retina (Fig. **113**).
2. The surface of the hamartoma classically shows a thickened, semi-translucent epiretinal membrane. Traction exerted by this membrane causes stress lines in the surrounding retina (cf. melanocytoma, *see* page 85).
3. Blood vessels coursing through the hamartoma are distorted and often dilated.
4. Combined hamartomas of the retina and RPE found in the peripheral retina are similar in appearance to those on the optic disc.

Supplementary findings

Combined hamartomas of the retina and RPE affecting the optic disc may be asymptomatic and discovered only on routine eye examination. The visual acuity is usually normal but the visual field shows an enlarged blind spot. Retinal traction does not usually develop until the fourth or fifth decade of life, when the patient may present with visual distortion. Retinal haemorrhage is a rare complication.

Combined hamartomas of the peripheral retina present at an earlier age (often in the first decade). Retinal traction is more severe and the visual acuity may be markedly reduced if the macula is affected—amblyopia and strabismus are then common findings.

Fluorescein angiography (Fig. **114**) demonstrates an abundant vascular supply and numerous dilated capillaries which may leak dye.

Associated systemic features

None known.

Differential diagnosis

A combined hamartoma of the retina and RPE has to be distinguished from:

1. Other pigmented lesions on the optic disc.
2. Other peripapillary pigmentary abnormalities.
3. Other lesions causing traction lines in the retina (e.g. persistent hyperplastic primary vitreous, proliferative diabetic retinopathy, *Toxocara canis*, retinopathy of prematurity).

113

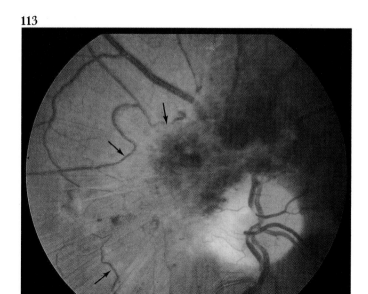

113 Combined hamartoma of the retina and RPE
extending from the superior margin of the optic disc.
Traction caused by the overlying, semi-transparent
epiretinal membrane has resulted in stress lines in the
surrounding retina. The adjacent retinal vessels are distorted
and dilated (arrows); some retinal haemorrhage has
occurred.

114

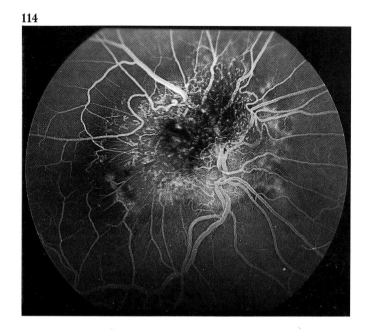

114 Fundus fluorescein angiogram of Fig. **113** showing
the abundant vascular supply and emphasizing the distorted,
dilated nature of the vessels.

Capillary haemangioma

A capillary haemangioma is a hamartoma composed of dilated blood vessels. It may be found either on the optic disc or in the peripheral retina.

Although it is a rare condition, capillary haemangioma of the optic disc is clinically important because of its relationship with haemangiomas of the retina and their possible systemic associations. About 50 per cent of patients with optic disc capillary haemangiomas also have retinal haemangiomas; these may be in the same eye, or in the contralateral eye. Patients who have a retinal haemangioma (with or without optic disc involvement) are said to have von Hippel's disease. Approximately half of those patients with a retinal capillary haemangioma also have haemangioblastomas of the cerebellum and viscera—this combination of features being known as von Hippel–Lindau disease (another of the phakomatoses; *see under* astrocytic hamartoma, page 87).

Ophthalmoscopy

Capillary haemangiomas of the optic disc exist in two morphologically distinct forms:

1. Typically, a localized, round, orange–pink vascular lesion is situated eccentrically on the disc and extends forwards into the vitreous, overlapping the disc margin; main branches of the retinal vessels may dip into the surface of the tumour (Fig. **115**).
2. Less frequently, a diffuse and indistinct flat, orange lesion extends from the optic disc into the adjacent retina.

Identification of a capillary haemangioma of the optic disc may be indicative of a haemangioma in the peripheral retina of the same eye, or even the fellow eye.

1. Retinal capillary haemangiomas are dome shaped and are often surrounded by extensive intraretinal exudate. There may be a related exaggerated macular response.
2. A peripheral retinal capillary haemangioma has a prominent feeding artery and draining vein extending from the optic disc to the retinal lesion; this is an important clinical clue (Fig. **116**). However, an early retinal

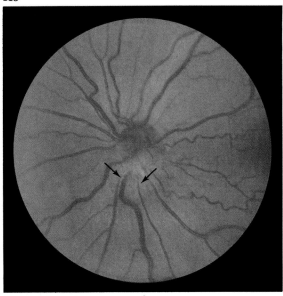

115 Capillary haemangioma of the optic disc. An orange lesion (arrows) is situated on the inferior half of the pink optic disc and extends into the retina. An enlarged retinal vein dips beneath its surface.

haemangioma may be difficult to locate ophthalmoscopically if the lesion (which resembles a pink macroaneurysm) is situated in the extreme periphery of the retina. Multiple lesions may be present in the same, or the fellow eye.

Supplementary findings

Capillary haemangiomas of the optic disc rarely increase in size, and then only slowly. Small retinal or vitreous haemorrhages may occur; these usually clear within a few months. Spontaneous sclerosis of the angioma has been described.

In contrast, progressive visual loss is common in cases of retinal capillary haemangioma and usually presents in the second decade. It is caused by an intraretinal accumulation of exudates leaking from the haemangioma; an exudative retinal detachment may result. Visual loss may also be caused by an exaggerated macular response (Fig. **117**), when exudates accumulate in this region, even though the

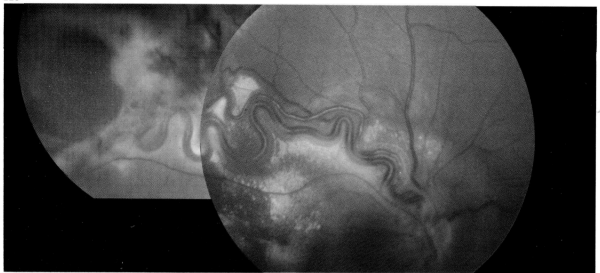

116 Retinal capillary haemangioma. A prominent feeding artery and draining vein extend between the optic disc and the dome-shaped lesion in the peripheral retina.

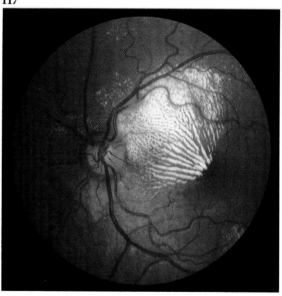

117 Exaggerated macular response with accumulation of exudates. A thorough examination of the peripheral retina is indicated in order to identify the causative lesion.

leaking haemangioma may be located some distance away in the peripheral retina. The presence of an exaggerated macular response should therefore prompt a thorough examination of the peripheral retina in order to identify its source. The reason why exudates accumulate preferentially at the site of the macula has not been established.

A capillary haemangioma of the retina is a progressive lesion which, because of chronic exudative retinal detachment, leads to secondary rubeosis of the iris, neovascular glaucoma and, eventually, phthisis of the eye. Thus patients with a capillary haemangioma require early referral for treatment. Retinal lesions may respond to laser photocoagulation or cryotherapy.

Associated systemic features

In von Hippel–Lindau disease, retinal capillary haemangiomas are associated with haemangioblastomas of the cerebellum and viscera, particularly the kidneys. This disease may be transmitted as an autosomal dominant trait with variable penetrance.

Differential diagnosis

Capillary haemangiomas of the optic disc have to be distinguished from other disorders:

1. Producing a hyperaemic, swollen disc.
2. Forming vascular masses on the optic disc.

The enlarged feeding and draining vessels of a peripheral retinal haemangioma require differentiation from other enlarged vessels extending from the optic disc.

Cavernous haemangioma

This is a rare hamartoma and involves the retinal venous system. It consists of clusters of thin-walled saccular venous aneurysms resembling bunches of grapes, usually situated in the retina, but occasionally affecting vessels on the optic disc. It almost always occurs unilaterally.

A few familial cases have been described, with associated systemic features; a dominant pattern of inheritance has been suggested.

Ophthalmoscopy

1. Grape-like saccular aneurysms (Fig. **118**) are seen lying flat on the retina; they may be partially covered by white gliotic or fibrous tissue.
2. Circulation through the haemangioma is sluggish and blood tends to stagnate in each saccule, with red blood cells sedimenting in response to gravity, leaving a pale layer of plasma above.

Supplementary findings

These haemangiomas are usually asymptomatic and may remain unchanged for many years. They very rarely leak fluid and even more rarely bleed; if leakage into the vitrous does occur, the blood usually clears spontaneously within a few weeks.

Fluorescein angiography shows an absolutely characteristic pattern. Transit time is slow and the saccules, hypofluorescent during the arterial phase, fill slowly during the venous phase, with the fluorescein pooling in the upper portion of each saccule.

Cavernous haemangiomas do not require treatment.

Associated systemic features

Although no definitive hereditary pattern has been established, some familial cases have been described in which vascular lesions, similar to those in the eye, occur in the skin and central nervous system. The use of computerized tomography may therefore be indicated for patients with ocular cavernous haemangiomas, to investigate for neural involvement.

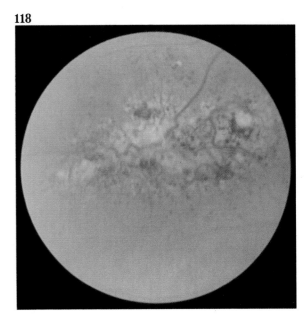

118

118 Cavernous haemangioma with grape-like venous aneurysms.

Differential diagnosis

This rare but very characteristic lesion can usually be identified with confidence and distinguished from other vascular masses on the optic disc.

Tumours arising from the optic nerve or its sheath

Glioma

Optic disc abnormalities arise in 90 per cent of patients with a glioma of the optic nerve. The disc abnormality usually takes the form of primary optic atrophy but, less commonly, the glioma may involve the disc itself.

The majority of cases (85 per cent) occur before the age of 20 years and more commonly in females than males. The presence of a glioma may be manifest at birth, but the tumour is most often diagnosed between the ages of 4 and 8 years, when it presents with unilateral proptosis. In children the glioma represents a relatively benign neoplasm, but in adults it is a much more malignant tumour, a glioblastoma.

Ophthalmoscopy

1. A glioma situated posteriorly to the lamina cribrosa may cause primary optic atrophy (*see* page 67).
2. A glioma of the optic disc consists of a smooth, elevated, white mass, partially or completely obscuring the disc (Fig. **119**).
3. Compression of the disc may cause occlusion of the central retinal vessels and their attendant complications (*see* pages 49, 51).

Supplementary findings

Proptosis may be the presenting feature (Fig. **120**), with limitation of ocular movement; at this stage visual acuity may be only slightly affected (cf. meningioma, *see* page 97). Further loss of vision results in an afferent pupillary defect. Severe proptosis gives rise to corneal exposure. Radiological investigations, including computerized tomography, help to delineate the position and extent of the tumour (Fig. **121**); enlargement of the optic foramen is a typical finding. Treatment is by surgical excision of the blind eye and as much of the length of the optic

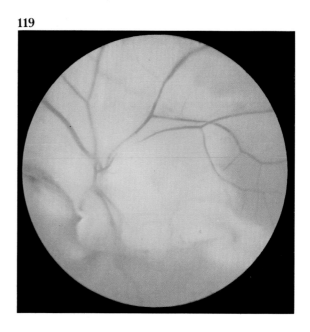

119

119 Glioma involving the optic nerve head. A rare presentation of optic nerve glioma.

nerve as is practicable. In adults, radiation therapy to the orbit may also be required.

Associated systemic features

Fifty-five per cent of patients with an optic nerve glioma can be expected to have neurofibromatosis and the patient should be examined for the ocular and systemic features of this syndrome (*see under* astrocytic hamartoma, page 87).

Differential diagnosis

Glioma of the optic nerve has to be differentiated from:

1. Other causes of primary optic atrophy.
2. Other conditions causing pale swellings on the optic disc.

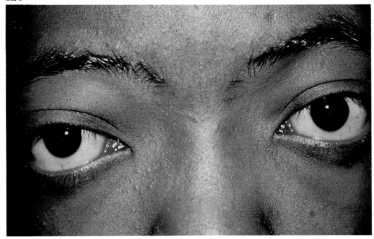

120 Proptosis of the right eye caused by an optic nerve glioma.

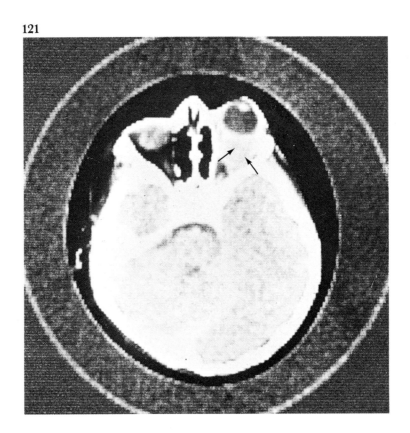

121 Computerized tomography scan showing an optic nerve glioma appearing as a retrobulbar mass (arrow) in the orbit.

Meningioma

A meningioma arises either from the meningeal sheaths surrounding the intraorbital optic nerve, or from a sphenoidal wing meningioma which extends into the orbit; its clinical manifestations reflect involvement of the optic nerve, either directly or as the result of compression.

Meningiomas show a bimodal distribution related to age: more than 50 per cent occur in patients over 30 years of age (typically white females) and more than 40 per cent in patients younger than 20 years, when it is a more progressive and lethal disorder. Meningiomas are occasionally reported in children under 2 years of age, raising the question whether—in this group at least—they are a congenital condition.

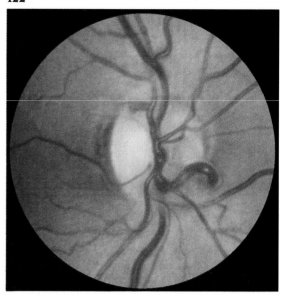

122 Opticociliary shunt vessel secondary to an optic nerve meningioma.

Ophthalmoscopy

A meningioma may present in one of two ways on ophthalmoscopy:

1. Rarely, there is direct involvement of the optic nerve, giving rise to an elevated, pale mass which obscures the optic disc and displaces the peripapillary retina. Splinter haemorrhages may be seen on the surface of the mass.
2. More commonly, the changes seen are those due to slow and progressive compression of the optic nerve behind the globe. These present as a triad of signs which are virtually pathognomic for meningioma, namely: (i) reduced visual acuity; (ii) a pale, swollen optic disc; and (iii) opticociliary shunt vessels (*see* below).

Supplementary findings

There is a characteristically early but slowly progressive loss of visual acuity. Compression of the central retinal vessels in the optic nerve leads to the development of opticociliary shunt vessels (Fig. **122**). These vessels divert blood from the optic disc into the peripapillary choroidal circulation (*see* page 56).

Proptosis is a late sign, only occurring when the tumour has extended outside the dura to form an enlarging mass behind the globe; it is therefore a difficult tumour to diagnose at an early stage in its development (cf. glioma, *see* page 95).

Treatment is by surgical excision of the tumour, although the intimate association between the dural sheath and the optic nerve makes this procedure hazardous.

Associated systemic features

Meningiomas of the optic nerve may occur as an isolated finding, or as a feature of neurofibromatosis (*see under* astrocytic hamartoma, page 87).

Differential diagnosis

The differential diagnosis depends upon the mode of presentation of the tumour:

1. When there is direct involvement of the optic nerve, a meningioma must be differentiated from other conditions showing a pale, swollen or distorted optic disc.
2. More commonly, a meningioma that compresses the retrobulbar portion of the optic nerve, resulting in the formation of an opticociliary shunt vessel, must be distinguished from other conditions associated with enlarged or abnormal vessels on the optic disc.

Tumours surrounding or extending into the optic disc

Retinoblastoma

Retinoblastoma is a congenital tumour, derived from neural elements in the primitive retina. It is the most common malignant intraocular tumour occurring in infants and children (1:15 000 live births) and about 30 per cent of patients are affected bilaterally; there may be several malignant foci in each eye. Although the tumours originate in the retina, the optic disc is subject to invasion (Fig. **123**) and its involvement is a very ominous sign, presaging intracranial spread of the malignancy.

The genetic determinants of the disorder are somewhat complex. In about 6 per cent of cases the condition is inherited as an autosomal dominant trait with incomplete penetrance. However, the majority of cases (94 per cent) appear to arise through sporadic mutation. One-quarter of these mutations may be transmitted to the next generation, but three-quarters are somatic mutations and do not affect the offspring of the patient. There is a 98 per cent chance that a patient with bilateral retinoblastoma represents a genetic mutation. Thus it is very difficult to make accurate predictions about likely inheritance patterns within a particular family, and hence to provide reliable genetic counselling.

Ophthalmoscopy

Two forms of tumour are described, namely exophytic and endophytic.

An exophytic tumour is flat and diffuse, extending into the subretinal space; it may be associated with a surrounding non-rhegmatogenous retinal detachment.

An endophytic tumour varies in appearance according to its stage of development:

1. At an early stage it forms a small, grey elevation with prominent overlying vasculature. Later the tumour becomes a raised, mushroom-shaped excrescence, creamy-pink in colour, with superficial telangiectatic

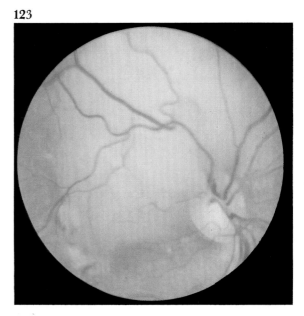

123 Retinoblastoma invading the optic disc. The overlying retinal vessels are prominent.

124 Retinoblastoma undergoing necrosis. The fundus view is hazy because of tumour debris in the vitreous.

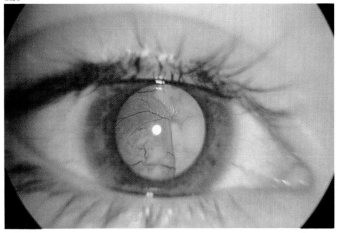

125 Leukocoria (cat's eye sign). The retinoblastoma, with dilated vessels on its surface, forms a pale mass behind the pupil.

126

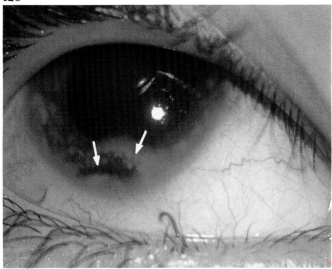

126 Retinoblastoma seeded in the anterior segment of the eye (arrows).

vessels and haemorrhages. A large draining vein may pass from the tumour to the optic disc. As the tumour outgrows its blood supply it undergoes necrosis and calcifies, so that its surface takes on a white, chalky appearance.

2. The vitreous is usually clear, but if seeding from the tumour takes place the vitreous may be filled with grey, feathery opacities. Necrosis of the tumour produces cellular debris in the vitreous (Fig. **124**).

3. One per cent of retinoblastomas regress spontaneously, leaving a fibrotic nodule, likely to be discovered during a routine fundus examination.

Supplementary findings

The majority of cases present around 18 months of age with leukocoria, loss of vision and a dilated, fixed pupil (cat's eye amaurosis, Fig. **125**). The next most common presenting sign is strabismus.

In addition, spread into the anterior segment of the eye (Fig. **126**) causes abnormalities of the iris which may include heterochromia, neovascularization and hyphaema. If spontaneous necrosis of the tumour takes place, the child may present with a sterile endophthalmitis.

Tumour spread to the brain may take place directly through the optic nerve, or indirectly via the subarachnoid space. Orbital invasion causes secondary proptosis. Metastases may pass to the viscera via the blood and lymphatics.

The highly vascular tumour is readily demonstrated by fundus fluorescein angiography; this technique may be helpful in the diagnosis of early exophytic tumours which may be difficult to identify ophthalmoscopically.

Seventy per cent of retinoblastomas contain calcium which shows up on ultrasonography, computerized tomography (Fig. **127**) and conventional radiology.

Treatment techniques include laser photocoagulation, cryotherapy, radiotherapy, or enucleation. Criteria for choice of technique are complex and management of these patients is best carried out at specialist centres.

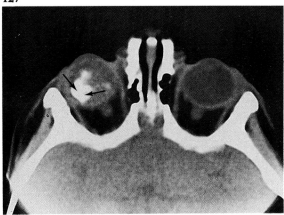

127 Computerized tomography scan showing a retinoblastoma as an intraocular, calcified mass (arrows).

Associated systemic features

These generally reflect disorders caused by metastases of the primary tumour, the most common sites being the brain and the liver. Sixteen per cent of those patients who survive bilateral retinoblastoma have been reported to develop an unrelated neoplasm later in life.

Differential diagnosis

1. A retinoblastoma invading the optic disc has to be distinguished from other conditions in which the optic disc is pale, swollen and distorted.

2. Retinoblastoma also has to be differentiated from other conditions presenting with leukocoria and strabismus, namely: the anterior form of persistent hyperplastic primary vitreous, retinopathy of prematurity (retrolental fibroplasia), congenital cataract and *Toxocara canis*.

Choroidal melanoma

Choroidal melanoma is the commonest primary intraocular malignancy occurring in adults. It arises in uveal tissue, most frequently in the choroid (80 per cent), but sometimes in the iris or ciliary body. Tumours situated anteriorly rarely involve the optic disc which may, however, be invaded by a choroidal melanoma situated posterior to the equator of the eye. The tumour may be either diffuse or circumscribed in form: the diffuse variety is the more invasive of the two and hence has a worse prognosis.

The condition is generally unilateral, usually occurring in patients aged over 50 years at the time of presentation; it is rarely found in children. Its distribution is almost completely restricted to whites (1:6000); only 1 per cent of melanomas are found in the coloured races (cf. melanocytoma, *see* page 85).

Ophthalmoscopy

1. The diffuse type of melanoma presents as a flat, plaque-like subretinal lesion, yellow-brown in colour. Those involving the optic disc are situated in the juxtapapillary region, the disc itself becoming swollen, hyperaemic and oedematous as a result of compression.
2. The circumscribed type of melanoma is a round, elevated outgrowth which may extend into the juxtapapillary region and optic disc (Fig. **128**). Its surface is typically mottled with grey, owing to pigment clumping; occasionally only a very small amount of pigment is present, when the lesion is known as an amelanotic melanoma.
3. An associated serous retinal detachment is a common finding; cystoid macular oedema may also occur.

Supplementary findings

Reduced visual acuity and visual field defects are common early findings.

Tumours in the posterior part of the eye are generally painless. Those that are anteriorly situated may present as a painful, blind eye, with compression of the drainage angle and secondary glaucoma. In cases where there is compression of the optic disc by a circum-

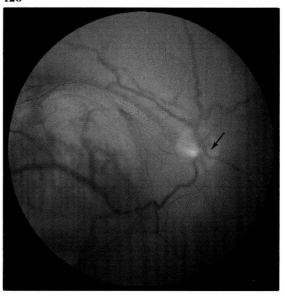

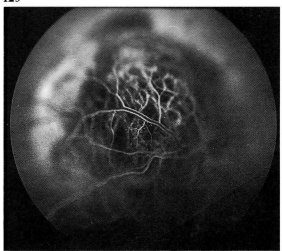

128 Choroidal melanoma. A large, raised tumour occupies the fundus. The optic disc (arrow) lies behind the plane of focus.

129 Fundus fluorescein angiogram of the eye shown in Fig. **128**. The highly vascular tumour shows early leakage of dye (cf. melanocytoma, Fig. **108**).

papillary tumour, retinal vein occlusion forms a rare complication (*see* page 51).

Extension of the tumour (particularly the diffuse type) may occur intracranially, either via the subarachnoid space, or along the optic nerve; scleral penetration with orbital invasion may cause proptosis.

Fundus fluorescein angiography (Fig. **129**) reveals a vascular, hyperfluorescent tumour which profusely leaks dye at the end stage of the angiogram (cf. melanocytoma, *see* page 85). In those patients in whom the fundus view is obscured, for example by the presence of a cataract, diagnosis may be assisted by the use of ultrasonography.

The management of choroidal melanoma is currently a subject of controversy. In cases of small tumours, observation is the most widely practised form of management, active intervention only being indicated with progression of the tumour. It is now thought that enucleation of the eye may promote metastatic spread and hence treatment modalities—such as photocoagulation, cryotherapy, radiation therapy, or local excision—tend to be favoured.

Choroidal osteoma (Osseous choristoma of the choroid)

A choristoma arises as a tumour-like mass of developmental origin, containing tissues foreign to the site from which it derives (cf. hamartoma, *see* page 87). Thus a choroidal osteoma represents an area of ossification in the choroid; it is often situated in the juxtapapillary region.

It is a very rare condition, occurring mainly in young females; there is no hereditary pattern.

Ophthalmoscopy

1. The optic disc may be of normal appearance or, if the tumour surrounds it, may show secondary swelling due to compression.
2. The tumour has an orange, mottled surface which shows a variable degree of pigmentary atrophy and clumping.
3. The margins of the tumour are irregular but sharply defined; they form pseudopodia and make a 'geographical', or map-like, pattern (Fig. **130**).
4. An abundant and plexiform network of choroidal vessels supplies the tumour, the disposition of the vessels being reminiscent of the Haversian canal system in true bone.
5. Associated findings on ophthalmoscopy may include subretinal neovascularization and haemorrhage with subsequent scar formation. Occasionally, a shallow exudative retinal detachment is present.

Associated systemic features

The highly malignant nature of the choroidal melanoma may cause the patient to present with metastases, particularly in the liver or the lungs.

Differential diagnosis

Choroidal melanoma has to be differentiated from other conditions presenting as pigmented swellings of the optic disc.

Supplementary findings

A choroidal osteoma gradually increases in size; if situated in the juxtapapillary region, gradual compression of the optic disc (Fig. **131**) leads to enlargement of the blind spot. Subretinal neovascularization and consequent disciform elevation of the retina may give rise to haemorrhage and sudden loss of vision. This complication may be suitable for treatment by laser photocoagulation.

The fluorescein angiogram is quite characteristic, showing a diffuse and mottled pattern of hyperfluorescence, again reminiscent of the Haversian canal system. The osteoma contains calcium and therefore shows up on radiology, computerized tomography and ultrasonography.

Associated systemic features

None known.

Differential diagnosis

Choroidal osteoma has to be distinguished from:

1. Other intraocular tumours surrounding the optic disc, as described in this chapter.
2. Other causes of peripapillary scarring.

Cases in which the optic disc is swollen require differentiation from those abnormalities associated with papilloedema.

130

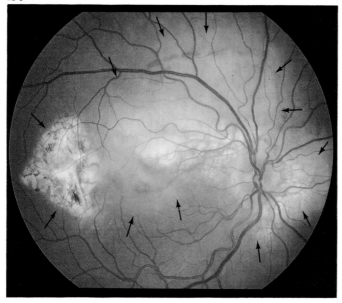

130 Choroidal osteoma. An orange–pink tumour surrounds the optic disc; its margin (arrows) has a map-like outline. The pale, triangular scar has resulted from previous subretinal neovascularization and haemorrhage.

131

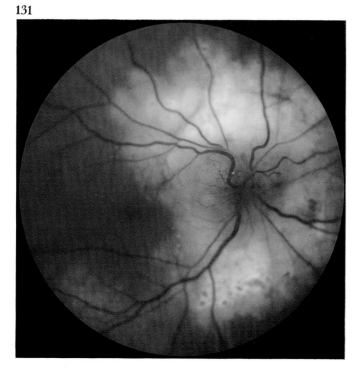

131 A swollen, congested optic disc, secondary to compression by a surrounding choroidal osteoma.

Metastases

These are probably the most common malignant tumours of the eye. Metastases to the eye occur from primary tumours situated in many of the viscera and endocrine glands, but most commonly from the breast in females and the lung in males. In 20 per cent of cases both eyes are involved.

The optic disc may be affected in various ways. Most frequently it is by extension of the tumour from the choroid to the optic disc (the choroid, being highly vascular, is a prime target site for metastases); less commonly the optic disc itself is the site of the metastasis. Alternatively, secondary changes in the optic disc may result from metastases in the retrobulbar portion of the optic nerve, or intracranially.

Ophthalmoscopy

1. A metastasis on the optic disc itself causes enlargement and distortion of the disc by the overlying yellow-white tumour mass.
2. Choroidal metastases present as pale, cream-coloured masses (Fig. **132**); they may occur independently, or with an optic disc metastasis in the same or the contralateral eye. An affected eye is likely to contain several lesions. The overlying retina may have a mottled, 'salt-and-pepper' appearance due to associated changes in the retinal pigment epithelium. A serous retinal detachment is a common finding.
3. If the optic disc is extensively ·affected, compression may cause retinal vein occlusion (*see* page 51).
4. Metastases posterior to the lamina cribrosa result in a variable appearance of the optic disc; retrobulbar compression of the optic nerve may lead to swelling of the optic disc and secondary optic atrophy (*see* page 68).
5. Papilloedema (*see* page 75) may be found when intracranial metastases are sufficiently extensive to cause raised intracranial pressure.

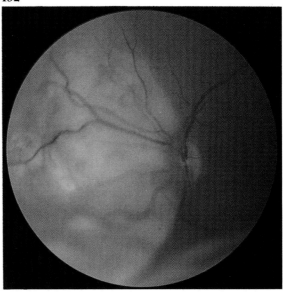

132 Choroidal metastasis extending onto the optic disc. The primary tumour was in the breast.

Supplementary findings

In 80 per cent of patients with metastases, reduced visual acuity is a presenting feature and visual field defects are common. Necrosis of the tumours may give rise to intraocular inflammation and secondary glaucoma. Orbital metastases or extraocular extension of the tumour may cause a painful proptosis and corneal exposure.

Associated systemic features

Associated systemic features are those of the primary tumour.

Differential diagnosis

1. Metastases on the optic disc have to be distinguished from other conditions in which the disc is pale, swollen and distorted.
2. Choroidal metastases have to be differentiated from other intraocular tumours surrounding the optic disc, described in this chapter.
3. The various causes of secondary optic atrophy or papilloedema may also have to be considered.

Leukaemic infiltrates

Many patients with leukaemia show ocular involvement, the acute form of the disease affecting the eye more commonly than the chronic form. Infiltration of the optic disc occurs in about one-third of cases and is of considerable clinical significance: its presence is related to active bone-marrow disease in the patient and therefore indicates that prompt and aggressive systemic treatment is required.

Although the optic disc is subject to direct metastatic spread, the vascular choroid is the structure most commonly infiltrated by leukaemic metastatic cells, with the optic disc subsequently being affected—a pattern similar to that occurring in cases of metastatic tumours (*see* page 104). Papilloedema is likewise a secondary manifestation of leukaemia, again resulting from raised intracranial pressure caused by central nervous system involvement. However, in cases of leukaemia, papilloedema may additionally be caused by iatrogenic factors, such as long-term treatment with high doses of systemic steroids.

Ophthalmoscopy

1. In the early stages of infiltration by leukaemic cells the optic disc appears pale, swollen and semi-opaque and its margin may be ill-defined (Fig. **133**).
2. At a later stage yellow deposits appear on the disc or retina (Fig. **134**) and there may be an accumulation of subretinal fluid in the juxtapapillary region, subsequent to destruction of the retinal pigment epithelium.
3. Retinal vessels are often sheathed.
4. Bone-marrow suppression may give rise to signs of severe anaemia (Fig. **135**), namely a pale fundus with arterioles and venules of similar colour; cotton-wool infarcts and retinal haemorrhages, typically with a white centre and dark periphery (Roth spots), may also occur. Associated platelet deficiency may cause preretinal and subhyaloid haemorrhages which may rupture into the vitreous.
5. Papilloedema or secondary optic atrophy is sometimes present.

133

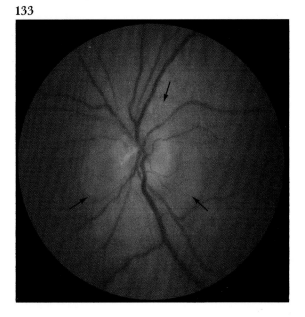

134

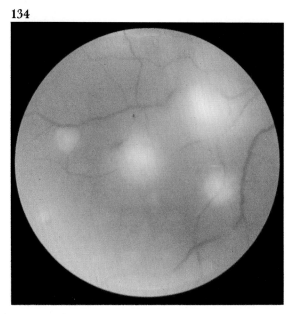

133 Leukaemic infiltration of the optic disc and surrounding retina (arrows); the margin of the optic disc is ill-defined.

134 Leukaemic deposits in the retina.

Supplementary findings

Intraocular infiltration invariably leads to irreversible loss of visual acuity and requires active intervention with systemic or local treatment (the latter by radiotheraphy). Other ocular features include painful proptosis, caused by orbital infiltration by leukaemic cells or haemorrhage into the orbital tissues. Cranial nerve infiltration results in ptosis and ophthalmoplegia.

Associated systemic features

Associated systemic features are those of the primary disorder.

Differential diagnosis

1. The differential diagnosis for intraocular leukaemic infiltrates is the same as that for intraocular metastases (*see* page 104).
2. Leukaemic infiltrates can usually be distinguished from metastases, however, by the ophthalmoscopic signs of severe anaemia and platelet deficiency which occur more commonly—although not exclusively—in leukaemia.

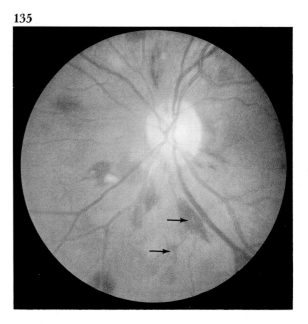

135 Fundus abnormalities in severe anaemia, secondary to leukaemia. There are numerous haemorrhages, cotton-wool infarcts and Roth spots (arrows); arterioles and venules are similar in colour.

8: Inflammatory Disorders

Granuloma of the optic disc

Granulomas of the optic disc may be associated with a uveitis affecting either the posterior pole (choroiditis) and/or the anterior segment of the eye (iritis). Recognition of an optic disc granuloma is clinically important, since it should alert to the possibility of an associated systemic disease and the need for its diagnosis.

The causes and associations of optic disc granulomas are numerous and include infective disorders (e.g. the parasitic infection, *Toxocara canis*) and granulomatous disorders (e.g. sarcoidosis). *Toxocara canis* most commonly affects children who are infected by ingesting eggs of the ascarid worm (by contamination from dog faeces); the larvae are disseminated from the gut to other viscera, including the eye. Sarcoidosis is a granulomatous disorder of uncertain aetiology which may affect almost any organ in the body.

Ophthalmoscopy

The ophthalmoscopic manifestations of a granuloma of the optic disc are similar, despite the varied aetiology of the primary disorders; appearances of the disc may be divided into those characteristic of the acute phase, and long-term changes.

In the acute phase (Fig. **136**):

1. There is a raised lesion affecting the optic disc and possibly extending into the adjacent retina; the lesion may be irregular in outline and quite hyperaemic.
2. Subretinal fluid accumulates around the optic disc, sometimes giving rise to an exudative retinal detachment in the peripheral retina.
3. Retinal blood vessels show evidence of phlebitis and vascular occlusion and haemorrhages may be seen in the retina.

136

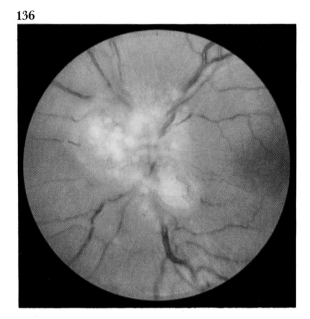

137

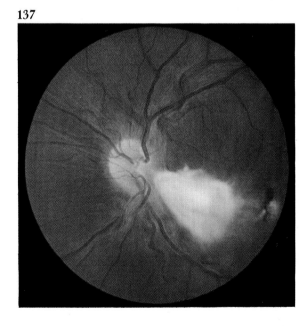

136 Inflammatory granuloma overlying the optic disc.

137 Granulomatous scar formation following infection by *Toxocara canis*. A white mass extends from the optic disc; there are traction lines in the nearby retina.

4. Ill-defined, pale areas of retinal infiltrate sometimes occur.
5. Exudates of inflammatory material accumulating in the vitreous often make the fundus view hazy.

In the later phases (Fig. **137**):

1. A white mass of scar tissue overlies the optic disc and causes traction retinal folds (a common feature of parasitic infection); leukocoria may occur.
2. Juxtapapillary scarring may also be present.
3. Sarcoidosis often shows the sequelae of retinovascular occlusion (*see* pages 49, 51).

Supplementary findings

Concomitant inflammation of the anterior segment of the eye gives rise to iritis and secondary glaucoma, the severity of which varies according to the primary aetiology. In cases of *Toxocara canis* the whole eye may become inflamed, causing endophthalmitis. In sarcoidosis, acute granulomatous anterior uveitis (iritis), with 'mutton fat' keratic precipitates on the cornea, are a common ocular manifestation. Lacrimal gland involvement may cause dry eyes (i.e. keratoconjunctivitis sicca — Sjögren's syndrome).

Associated systemic features

These relate to the systemic disorder.

Differential diagnosis

Granulomas of the optic disc:

1. During the acute stage, have to be distinguished from other conditions in which the optic disc is hyperaemic and swollen.
2. During the later stages, have to be distinguished from other conditions in which the optic disc is pale and distorted.
3. At the end stage, have to be distinguished from other conditions causing juxtapapillary scarring.

Juxtapapillary choroiditis

In juxtapapillary choroiditis, also known as Jensen's choroiditis (Fig. **138**), focal patches of inflammation arise in close proximity to the optic nerve head. The condition is particularly a manifestation of two systemic disorders: in developed countries it is most likely to result from infection by the protozoan parasite *Toxoplasma gondii*, whereas tuberculosis is the most probable causal agent in those areas where the disease remains endemic.

Toxoplasmosis is usually a congenital condition, transmitted from mother to conceptus during the first trimester of pregnancy, when the developing eyes are invariably affected. However, early lesions generally heal when the parasites become encysted and only retinochoroidal scarring is found on routine fundus examination. Recurrence may occur, following the liberation of encysted organisms and evoking further damage to the retina as the result of an immune response.

Tuberculosis, like toxoplasmosis, shows chorioretinal involvement; recognition of a case of juxtapapillary choroiditis should therefore be followed by prompt referral for confirmatory diagnosis of the causal agent.

Ophthalmoscopy

(i) Toxoplasmosis

In the acute phase:

1. This infection presents with a white, necrotizing retinochoroiditis, having the appearance of an ill-defined, white lesion which may extend from the optic disc itself, or be situated in the nearby retina. The presence of such a lesion should prompt a thorough examination of the fundus for further, satellite lesions.
2. The vitreous may appear hazy and contain inflammatory cells.

In the later stage:

1. There are typical atrophic scars (Fig. **139**) in the juxtapapillary retina, irregular in outline and having a pigmented margin.
2. Pallor of the optic disc occurs in that segment related to the retinal changes; it is caused by nerve fibre loss.

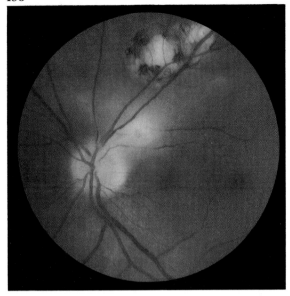

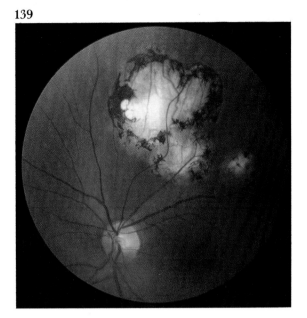

138 Jensen's choroiditis. There is an ill-defined, pale area of juxtapapillary inflammation. A satellite atrophic scar with a pigmented border is evidence of a previous episode of infection.

139 Toxoplasmosis. Necrotizing retinochoroiditis has resulted in an atrophic scar with an irregular but well-defined pigmented border.

(ii) Tuberculosis

In the acute phase:

This infection may similarly present with an ill-defined, pale lesion in the juxtapapillary region. Detailed examination of the fundus may reveal numerous, scattered tubercles. Rarely, a large, solitary tuberculoma may be found.

In the later stage:

The juxtapapillary scar may be indistinguishable from that found in toxoplasmosis; in tuberculosis, however, scars in the peripheral fundus remain distinct and do not coalesce.

Supplementary findings

Visual loss may be severe and progressive owing to the intimate relationship between the juxtapapillary choroiditis and the optic nerve head. Visual impairment may also be brought about by the presence of inflammatory cells in the vitreous. Evidence of anterior segment inflammation (iritis) may be found.

Associated systemic features

Those related to the primary disorder.

Differential diagnosis

Cases of juxtapapillary choroiditis:

1. In the acute stage, have to be distinguished from other conditions in which the optic disc appears pale and distorted.
2. In the late stage, have to be distinguished from other conditions showing peripapillary scarring and/or other peripapillary pigmentary abnormalities.

9: Other Peripapillary Abnormalities

Two rare disorders—angioid streaks and serpiginous choroidopathy—are considered in this chapter. Their grouping is purely a matter of convenience; the two conditions are unrelated and, as far as is known, the pathological manifestations of each occur only in the retina or choroid and are not preceded by, or associated with, degenerative changes in the optic disc. However, both disorders are anatomically intimately related to the optic disc. They are therefore easily discernible during routine ophthalmoscopy, and their discovery should prompt detailed examination of both fundi.

Angioid streaks of the retina

Angioid streaks take the form of grey-brown lesions emanating from around the margin of the optic disc and radiating in the retina. They arise as a result of breaks in Bruch's membrane, caused by defects in elastic and collagenous tissues. Affected eyes are especially vulnerable to trauma; subretinal neovascularization, with haemorrhage and scarring, may permanently impair visual acuity.

Although occurring as an independent ocular finding in 50 per cent of cases, the presence of angioid streaks should also alert to the possibility of an associated systemic disease. They may occur in inherited connective-tissue disorders, such as the Grönblad–Strandberg syndrome and the Ehlers–Danlos syndrome, as well as in other conditions (*see* below).

Ophthalmoscopy

(Figs. **140, 141**)

1. There are grey-brown streaks, of irregular width and outline, which radiate from an area of peripapillary atrophy.
2. Angioid streaks branch in a manner similar to that of the retinal vessels they also taper peripherally. However, the fact that they lie underneath the vessels provides a distinguishing feature.
3. There may be macular involvement, with retinal haemorrhage or scar formation.
4. The peripheral fundus sometimes shows stippled pigmentary change.
5. Optic disc drusen may be an associated finding.

Supplementary findings

The patient is asymptomatic until the complications associated with subretinal neovascularization develop. The effect on visual acuity is related to the extent and nature of the complications; if macular involvement progresses slowly the patient is likely to present with blurred vision, but haemorrhage into the macula precipitates sudden visual loss. The resultant macular scarring may then lead to a permanent central scotoma. These complications most often occur during the fourth decade of life and, although the condition is progressive, a plateau is usually reached around 55–60 years of age, after which vision remains fairly stable.

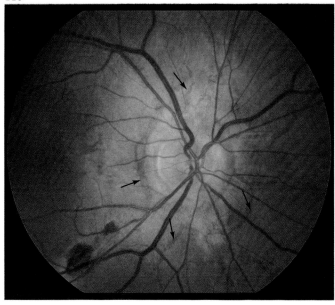

140 Angioid streaks (arrows) radiating from an area of peripapillary atrophy. The angioid streaks underlie the retinal blood vessels.

141

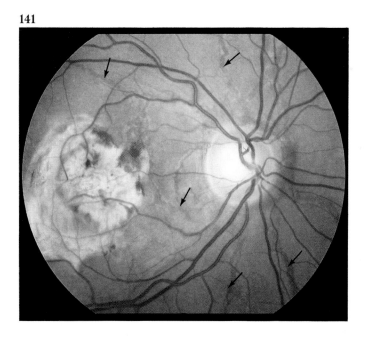

141 Angioid streaks (arrows) with an atrophic macular scar showing a residual haemorrhage.

142 Pseudoxanthoma elasticum. These xanthoma-like papular lesions occur on flexor surfaces and invariably affect the neck. With angioid streaks, they form the Grönblad–Strandberg syndrome.

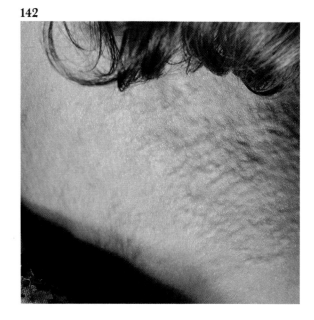

142

Associated systemic features

These are related to the underlying systemic disorder. In the Grönblad–Strandberg syndrome there are accompanying deficiencies in the elastic tissue of the skin (pseudoxanthoma elasticum, Fig. **142**) and arterial vascular tree. The latter may result in visceral or intracranial haemorrhage. In the Ehlers–Danlos syndrome, hyperelasticity of the skin and joints commonly occurs, with recurrent dislocations. Other systemic diseases occurring in association with angioid streaks include Paget's disease, acromegaly, sickle-cell anaemia, hypercalcaemia and lead poisoning.

Differential diagnosis

Angioid streaks have to be differentiated from other conditions in which there is peripapillary scarring.

Serpiginous choroidopathy

This condition (also called geographic helicoid peripapillary choroidopathy) consists of a progressive destruction of the retinal pigment epithelium and choriocapillaris. The lesions usually commence at the margin of the optic disc and extend, like snail tracks, towards the macula and mid-peripheral fundus.

The aetiology is unknown, although it is associated with ocular inflammation. Serpiginous choroidopathy usually affects adults in middle age and is bilateral, although often developing asymmetrically; the condition is untreatable and there is progressive and severe loss of vision. Early diagnosis and counselling may help the patient, assisting the adjustment of working and living patterns in anticipation of future visual handicap.

Ophthalmoscopy

In the acute stage:

Irregular, geographical areas of oedema affect the retinal pigment epithelium and choroid; the pale, oedematous lesions (Fig. **143**) extend in the manner of snail tracks from the optic disc towards the macula and mid-periphery of the fundus; isolated patches of degeneration ('skip areas') may also occur.

In the later stages:

1. The geographical pattern of distribution of the lesions increases in extent, while 'punched-out' pale scar tissue, representing areas of atrophy, form within the previously oedematous 'snail tracks'. Patches of hyperpigmentation appear at the margins of the scars (Fig. **144**).
2. Associated sub-retinal neovascularization and haemorrhage may result in further scar formation.
3. Retinal vessels overlying scar tissue may show signs of vasculitis.
4. Inflammatory cells may be seen in the vitreous, and rarely there may be an exudative retinal detachment.

Supplementary findings

Visual acuity is affected progressively, over a period of about 5 years; if the macula is affected, severe visual loss is the invariable outcome.

An associated mild anterior uveitis (iritis) occasionally occurs.

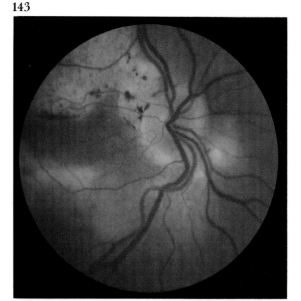

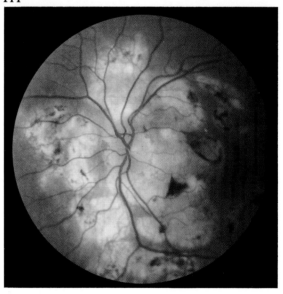

143 Serpiginous choroidopathy. Pale oedematous lesions extend from the optic disc towards the macula.

144 Serpiginous choroidopathy; a more advanced case showing scarring throughout the posterior pole of the fundus.

Associated systemic features
None known.

Differential diagnosis

Serpiginous choroidopathy has to be differentiated from other conditions in which there is peripapillary scarring.

Index